Commissioning for Health and Social Care

Institute of Public Care

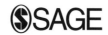

SAGE

Los Angeles | London | New Delhi
Singapore | Washington DC

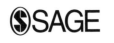

Los Angeles | London | New Delhi
Singapore | Washington DC

SAGE Publications Ltd
1 Oliver's Yard
55 City Road
London EC1Y 1SP

SAGE Publications Inc.
2455 Teller Road
Thousand Oaks, California 91320

SAGE Publications India Pvt Ltd
B 1/I 1 Mohan Cooperative Industrial Area
Mathura Road
New Delhi 110 044

SAGE Publications Asia-Pacific Pte Ltd
3 Church Street
#10-04 Samsung Hub
Singapore 049483

Editor: Alex Clabburn
Assistant editor: Emma Milman
Production editor: Katie Forsythe
Copyeditor: Chris Bitten
Indexer: Silvia Benvenuto
Marketing manager: Tamara Navaratnam
Cover design: Naomi Robinson
Typeset by: C&M Digitals (P) Ltd, Chennai, India
Printed in Great Britain by
CPI Group (UK) Ltd, Croydon, CR0 4YY

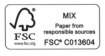

MIX
Paper from
responsible sources
FSC
www.fsc.org   FSC® C013604

First published 2014

Library of Congress Control Number: 2014933588

British Library Cataloguing in Publication data

A catalogue record for this book is available from the British Library

ISBN 978-1-4462-4924-6
ISBN 978-1-4462-4925-3 (pbk)

Contents

Acknowledgements

The Institute of Public Care (IPC) at Oxford Brookes University was established in 1987. It exists to promote well run evidence based public care. Commissioning, procurement and market facilitation in health and social care are key areas of practice for the Institute. The chapters in the book were written by a group of staff and Fellows at IPC and captures the learning from knowledge-transfer activities including consulting, research and teaching over those years. They are intended to be read as standalone chapters within a common overall framework, and as a result we include overlapping tools and ideas. IPC is very grateful to the many people we have worked with over the years from the National Health Service, local authorities and providers of care from the private, voluntary and non-for-profit sectors, as without them this book would not have been possible.

Professor Keith Moultrie, Director, Institute of Public Care

All of the members of the Institute of Public Care's team have contributed towards this book through their work on projects, teaching and writing since 1987. Thanks in particular to the following colleagues who have led for us in the writing of the chapters in the book:

- Juliet Bligh
- Professor John Bolton
- Katy Burch
- Liz Cairncross
- Dr Kam Dhillon
- Asa Johnsson Humphries
- Professor Andrew Kerslake
- Paul McGloin
- Steve Merell
- Professor Keith Moultrie
- Kathryn Rhodes

Publisher's Acknowledgements

Fig 1.2: NHS Information Centre commissioning cycle is republished with the permission of The Health and Social Care Information Centre.

Fig 1.3: National Audit Office (NAO) model of commisioning and civil society is republished with permission of the National Audit Office. To find out more visit nao.org.uk.

Fig 3.8: Locating priorities is republished with permission of Karen Newbigging and Chris Heginbotham.

1

An Introduction to Commissioning and Procurement

The 2008 financial crisis precipitated the world's deepest recession since the 1929 Wall Street Crash. Perhaps not surprisingly a consequence of the financial fallout was for governments to seek to reduce expenditure and maximise efficiency in their public services, while at the same time addressing the future additional demands presented by rises in demographics and service expectations. Many have turned to more effective commissioning and procurement to help them with this challenge. Yet what constitutes commissioning and procurement is often surrounded by mystery and half-truths; often the target of media criticism and widely misunderstood by the population. The aim of this book is to:

- de-mystify commissioning and procurement in health and social care;
- present methods and tools to carry out essential analytic activities for evidence-based intelligent commissioning decisions; and
- promote mature business practice in health and social care organisations, bringing together commissioners and service providers to offer choice and high quality outcomes for consumers.

This book is for new and established practitioners who commission and procure health, public health and social care services. It is a book that health and social practitioners can apply to business problems whatever their role in commissioning and procurement. It comprises a collection of separate papers which cover different aspects of the commissioning cycle so that some themes and ideas overlap. It is a practical guide and aid to practice rather than a theoretical discussion of the relative merits of commissioning, the market or private sector provision of public care services. Each chapter contains definitions, case-studies, exercises and 'stop and reflect' sections designed to provide knowledge and opportunities for the reader to engage with their own commissioning problems.

Commissioning represents a series of activities which together constitute a systematic approach to planning and resourcing public services. As such, it is up to practitioners to determine how best they can organise and apply commissioning activities to help deliver better services and ultimately better outcomes for the people they serve. Delivering value for money and building social capital and investment will be key drivers in the communities they serve.

In de-mystifying commissioning and procurement of public services, none of the activities involved are new or exclusive to specialist commissioners. In many ways they are simply activities that anyone involved in good management and business practice should be doing. Commissioning, now more than ever, require a focus on the balance of services across a market, and because of this focus, an evidence-based and systematic approach.

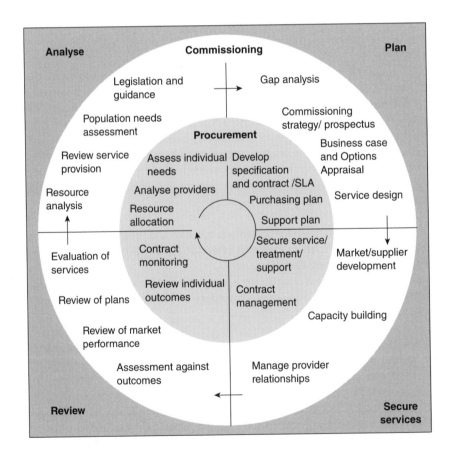

The Institute of Public Care (IPC) has reviewed many models of commissioning and procurement. This chapter presents the IPC model, which has developed over the last 10 years and forms the road map for the rest of this book. It is then split into four sections each containing three chapters of focused activities. Section 1 – Analyse – explores 'Why, When and How to Commission' in Chapter 2 and 'Conducting Strategic Needs Assessments' and 'Mapping Resources' in Chapters 3 and 4. Section 2 – Plan – covers 'Strategic Analysis Tools for Commissioning' and 'Managing the Strategy and Communicating with Stakeholders' in Chapters 5 and 6, followed by Chapter 7 that explores 'Towards Effective Service Design'. Section 3 – Secure Services – starts with Chapter 8 that presents how to conduct 'Market Facilitation' which has become a key component of the commissioning and procurement role today. This is followed by 'Procurement and the Contracting Process' and 'Contracting for Personalised Services' in the twenty-first century in Chapters 9 and 10 respectively. Section 4 – Review – covers three key areas of current interest: 'Managing Service Performance', 'Decommissioning' and 'Achieving Value for Money' in Chapters 11, 12 and 13 respectively.

Defining commissioning

The British Government's Modernising Commissioning Green Paper (Cabinet Office, 2011) defined commissioning as:

> The cycle of assessing the needs of people in an area, designing and then achieving appropriate outcomes. The service may be delivered by the public, private or civil society sectors.

Developing this perspective further, the Commissioning Support Programme (2009) defined commissioning as:

> The process for deciding how to use the total resource available for children, young people and parents and carers in order to improve outcomes in the most efficient, effective, equitable and sustainable way.

Commissioning represents a broad concept with many definitions. Most definitions of commissioning paint a picture of a cycle of activities at a strategic level – concerned with populations – including:

- assessing the needs of a population;
- setting priorities and developing plans to meet those needs in line with local and national targets;
- securing services from providers to meet those needs and targets through building mature relationships;

- monitoring and evaluating outcomes; and
- the above combined with an explicit requirement to consult and involve service users in the process.

Commissioning is much more than just contracting and procurement; crucially it involves a whole range of services, not just the contracts or agreements, with external suppliers. This often involves the use of a wide range of resources across local partners, i.e. the whole local system of cooperation between partners, including local authority services, Clinical Commissioning Groups and other health bodies, schools and colleges, youth justice agencies and others. These need to be deployed in the best way possible to improve outcomes.

Commissioners then are not just those with 'commissioning' in their job title but everyone who contributes to the commissioning process.

Defining procurement

Procurement is not the same as commissioning, although it is often used interchangeably. Procurement, purchasing and contracting are activities that focus on a specific part of the wider commissioning process – the selection, negotiation and agreement with the provider of what service is to be supplied. To be more specific:

- Procurement or purchasing usually refers to the process of finding and deciding on a provider and buying a service.
- Contracting usually refers to the negotiation and letting of a contract and its subsequent monitoring: formalising the purchasing process, including writing down want is wanted (spec) and how you will be paid etc. (contract), working out the relationship with the provider and the monitoring of their performance.

Procurement uses the contracting process to achieve effective commissioning here, but it is not the only activity available to commissioners to enable them to secure service improvements. There are alternative tools as well, such as influencing external organisations to focus their resources on achieving the outcomes you would like to see delivered through constructive dialogue, revising business plans, or redesigning existing internal or external services.

Multi-level commissioning and procurement

Commissioning is practised on different scales or 'levels'. There is not a single 'ideal' location for commissioning. The management task is to decide what is the most appropriate level to achieve the required outcomes, and hence the

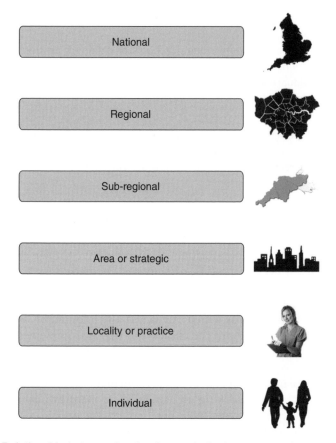

Figure 1.1   Relationship between levels of commissioning

specific local commissioning configuration, i.e. where to allocate the responsibility for carrying out particular commissioning activities. Different services require commissioning at different levels, depending on factors such as volume, maturity of the local market and provider relationships, safeguarding and risk, and price.

In every local area commissioners are therefore likely to undertake multi-level commissioning – commissioning at a mixture of levels to suit the needs of different services and populations.

Examples of the different levels of health and social care commissioning include:

- National and Regional – Highly specialist commissioning, e.g. national services for people with rare and complex conditions.
- Sub-regional, e.g. Pan-London Commissioning for sexual health services.

- Strategic – commissioning across the whole local area involving a range of partners, e.g. Total Place initiatives.
- Locality – Practice-based commissioning, schools or children's centres, or locality area-based commissioning.
- Individual – Individual budgets and direct payments, care and case management and budget-holding lead professional.

In recent years there has been an increased focus on service users and carers assuming the lead role in commissioning services to meet their own individual needs and aspirations (e.g. Direct Payments and Individual Budgets).

The commissioning and procurement cycles

There are many models of commissioning, but most have similar characteristics in that they describe a cyclical process of activities encompassing population needs assessment, aligning resources to meet needs, developing or purchasing services, and monitoring performance.

In many ways it matters less which one is actually adopted by local partners so long as there is agreement about the choice and that it is implemented well.

Many areas have adopted joint or integrated commissioning processes for service specific areas, e.g. for young people with mental health problems, people with substance-misuse problems. These arrangements tend to vary in terms of the degree to which joint-working and integration manifest, usually dependent on the maturity of relationships, whether budgets get pooled, or whether partners are co-located and use shared methods and resources.

Five models are presented here, followed by the IPC commissioning and procurement cycle which forms the road map for this book.

A general National Health Service model

The NHS model uses nine elements within three broader stages – strategic planning, procuring services, and monitoring and evaluation. Further information can be downloaded from the NHS Information Centre for Health and Social Care website at www.ic.nhs.uk/commissioning.

The NAO model

This NAO model highlights those elements of the commissioning cycle where they think that a good relationship with civil society organisations (CSOs) has a significant impact on helping commissioners achieve good value for money.

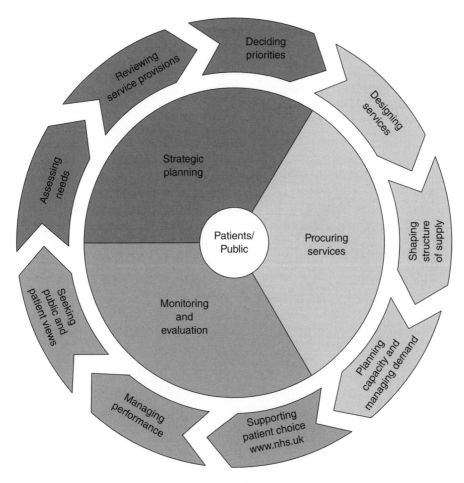

Figure 1.2 NHS Information Centre commissioning cycle

The local area model

Some local areas and regions have developed their own version of the commissioning and procurement process. The county of Essex has developed a steering wheel to describe their strategic commissioning process – as it moves back and forth rather than cyclically! (You can read more about this model at their website at www.socialfinance.org.uk/sites/default/files/vulnerable%20people%20essex%20 works_0.pdf).

Their model focuses on a multi-agency commissioning process, gaining agreement from all agencies. Key factors in their model are:

- Assessing needs and identifying priorities.
- Involving service users in the decision making process.
- Aligning with national priorities.
- Determining the full extent of available resources from all appropriate organisations.
- Monitoring delivery performance.
- Managing contracts and sourcing providers.
- Ensuring effective delivery, decommissioning and reshaping.

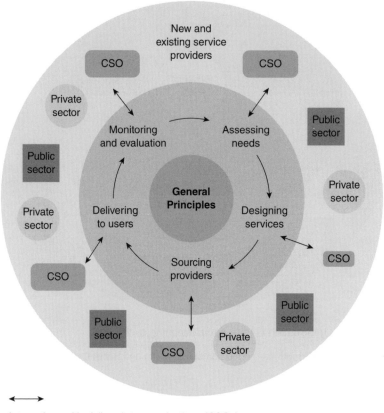

Interactions with civil society organisations (CSOs)

Figure 1.3   National Audit Office (NAO) model of commissioning and civil society

Source: National Audit Office. To findout more please visit nao.org.uk

The Commissioning Support Programme (CSP) model

The CSP approach was developed by the Springboard Consortium for the Department for Education in 2010 for children's services but is simple to use and consistent with other approaches and cycles.

The CSP model has a four-stage approach: understand, plan, do and review. The key principle here are that any commissioning cycle should start with understanding the outcomes that are being desired. Commissioners should actively seek to involve service users at each commissioning stage so that they become co-designers and co-producers of the positive outcomes which commissioning is striving to achieve. Service providers should also be involved at all stages. Other activities in the four stages include:

1. **Understand** – Recognise local outcomes, needs, resources and priorities and agree what the desired end product should be. This involves gathering the views of service users so that services can be configured most appropriately to address those needs within available resources. Providers are a key source of information and insight in this phase. Their views of the needs of children, young people and families should be considered, as well as their insight into what types of services and service configuration may be most appropriate in response. This should take into account – and inform – other needs assessment processes, for example the joint strategic needs assessment (JSNA).

2. **Plan** – Map out and consider different ways of addressing the needs identified through the needs assessment above. How can they be addressed effectively, efficiently, equitably and in a sustainable way? This way optimal use can be made of available resources regardless of who invests them. Providers should be involved at this stage particularly to add their expertise to the discussion. Plans need not just be about which service to use, but also the workforce and facilities.

3. **Secure Services** – Make decisions based on the appropriate action identified in the 'plan' stage to secure better outcomes using the resources available in the most efficient way.

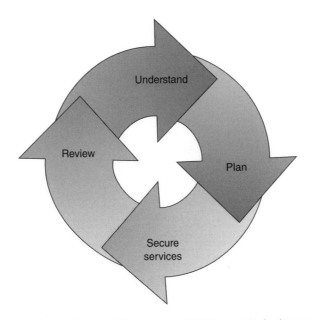

Figure 1.4 Commissioning Support Programme (CSP) commissioning cycle

This may be in full partnership or informal cooperation with individual partners undertaking activities aligned within the agreed plan.

4. **Review** – Monitor service delivery against expected outcomes and report how well
    it is performing against the plan. This is in effect asking – did our 'do' phase deliver
    on the 'plan' we put in place to deliver against what we 'understand' to be the needs?
    Then establish review commissioning arrangements to ensure the plan is working
    effectively.

The Office of Government Commerce model

The Office of Government Commerce (OGC), on its website, publishes a procurement process, which shows the stages involved in planning and managing a
generic procurement project (www.ogc.gov.uk/policy_and_standards_frame-
work_general_temp.asp). Procurement also follows a cycle, starting with the
identification of need to purchase a service and ending with the end of a contract, with at its centre Project and Programme Management and Risk
Management. This model also has similarities with the cyclical process of
commissioning.

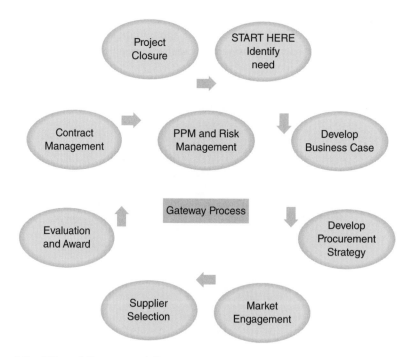

Figure 1.5 Office of Government Commerce: procurement process

The Institute of Public Care commissioning model

The IPC cycle, first developed in 2003 and since adapted, was adopted by Department of Communities and Local Government in their Guide to Procuring Care and Support Services (available at: www.spkweb.org.uk/Subjects/Capacity_ building/Procurement+guide+templates.htm). The IPC cycle shows the relationship between strategic commissioning (the outer circle), and procurement and individual commissioning (the inner circle). This cycle will form the road map for this book with four key sections: analyse, plan, do/secure services and review.

This IPC approach has been used widely by a variety of public bodies as it integrates commissioning with procurement, purchasing and contracting, and is a performance management methodology with a clear cycle of activities.

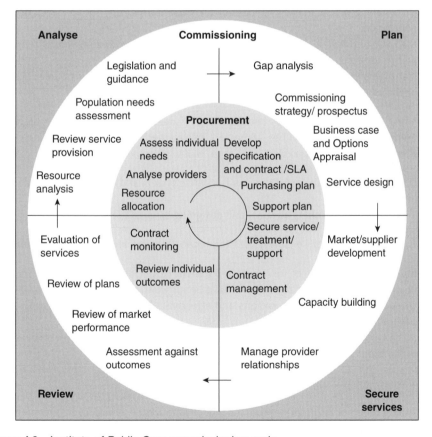

Figure 1.6   Institute of Public Care commissioning cycle

The key principles underpinning the IPC approach include:

- Activities are grouped into four elements and all four elements of the cycle are sequential and equally important.
- The commissioning and procurement cycles are linked; activities in one must inform the ongoing development of the other.
- The commissioning process must be equitable and transparent, and open to influence from all stakeholders via an on-going dialogue with patients/service users and providers.

The strategic commissioning activities identified in the outer circle include:

Analysis – understanding the values and purpose of the agencies involved, the needs they must address, and the environment in which they operate. This involves activities such as:

- Clarifying the priorities, and the research and best practice basis for the services.
- Undertaking needs analysis to identify the current and likely future needs of the population.
- Mapping and reviewing services across agencies to understand provider strengths and weaknesses.
- Identifying the resources currently available and agreeing future resources across agencies.

Planning – identifying the gaps between what is needed and what is available, and planning how these gaps will be addressed. This element of the commissioning cycle involves activities such as:

- Undertaking a gap analysis to review the whole system and identify what is needed in the future.
- Writing a commissioning strategy and designing services to meet needs.

Doing/securing services – ensuring that the services needed are delivered as planned:

- Managing the balance of services to reduce risk, i.e. deciding which services should be undertaken in-house and which should be sub-contracted from other providers.
- Developing good communications and effective relationships with existing and potential providers.
- Purchasing new services and de-commissioning services that do not meet the needs of the client group.

Reviewing – monitoring the impact of services:

- Pulling together information from individual contracts or service level agreements.
- Developing systems to bring together relevant data on finance, activity and outcomes to review the overall impact of services.

The procurement activities (inner circle) follow the same pattern of **analyse, plan, secure services** and **review** and consist of similar activities, but at a different level. Activities in the purchasing and SDS cycle include:

- Assessing users' needs and the strengths and weaknesses of providers, as well as the direction set in the commissioning strategy.
- Allocation of resources.
- Developing service specifications and deciding on contract type and terms.
- Developing and agreeing support plans.
- Day-to-day care and contract management and communication with providers.
- Securing support via Direct Payments.
- Tendering for services and letting of contracts.
- Monitoring and reviewing contracts and support plans.

A key starting point in effective commissioning is to ensure all local partners and key stakeholders have a shared vision for commissioning and procurement in order:

- to promote agreement to and understanding of the commissioning process and,
- that the process covers some form of needs analysis and planning, investment against this plan and review of the efficacy of the investment.

Ask yourself what needs to be done in your local area to develop a shared vision that can lead to high performing commissioning and procurement behaviours?

EXERCISE 1.1

Review the commissioning process for a particular population group, e.g. young adults with a learning disability, people with mental health problems.

Using the commissioning model, map the activities needed to ensure the effective commissioning of services to meet the needs of that group. Specify the roles and responsibilities of the people involved in this process.

EXERCISE 1.2

Governance

Governance is about systems of decision making, and the expectations for various roles and responsibilities that hold together the commissioning process. Governance arrangements should set out clearly for everyone involved who the individuals, groups and boards who are responsible for the various activities, tasks and stages of strategic commissioning. What enables effective governance?

- A strong planning process, with plans that are clearly linked through a 'golden thread'.
- A clear decision-making process within and across 'directorates'.
- A mutually adopted approach to commissioning, e.g. a commissioning framework.
- Development of local commissioning principles.
- Clarity of roles and responsibilities.

For example, if you are based in a local area in England, your governance arrangements might include:

Local Strategic Partnership	Community Plan	**What** do we want to achieve in the whole local area, for the whole population?
Health and Well-being Board	Health and wellbeing (HWB) strategy and Joint Strategic Needs Assessment (JSNA)	**What** are our health and wellbeing priorities? Is the JSNA the voice of the community?
Management Team	Commissioning framework	**How** are we going to run the commissioning function? What is our overall approach, boundaries, process and principles?
Commissioning Unit – Integrated/ Joint	Commissioning strategies and Market Position Statements	**How** are we going to meet the intentions and priorities set out in the H&WB Strategy, using the Commissioning Framework? What are our current and future supply issues and how are we going to need to respond?

Figure 1.8   An example of strategies, frameworks, plans and statements

Stop and Reflect

- What is the nature of your commissioning governance structures and processes?
- How could they be improved?
- How do you assess the impact you are making by your commissioning decisions to the population you serve?

Further reading and web-based resources

Department of Health (2009) *Securing Better Health for Children and Young People Through World Class Commissioning*. London: DH Publications.
Department of Health and Department for Children, Schools and Families (2009) *Healthy Lives, Brighter Futures: The Strategy for Children and Young People's Health*. Didcot: Health Protection Agency.

National Audit Office Available at: www.nao.org.uk/sectors/third_sector/successful_commissioning/successful_commissioning/introduction/nao_model_of_commissioning_and.aspx

Primary Care Commissioning Available at: www.pcc.nhs.uk/new-commissioning-resources

NHS Information Centre Commissioning Cycle. Available at: www.ic.nhs.uk/commissioning

IPC Available at: http://ipc.brookes.ac.uk/

Commissioning Support Programme Available at: www.commissioningsupport.org.uk www.gov.uk/government/news/modernising-commissioning-green-paper-published

Section 1

Analyse

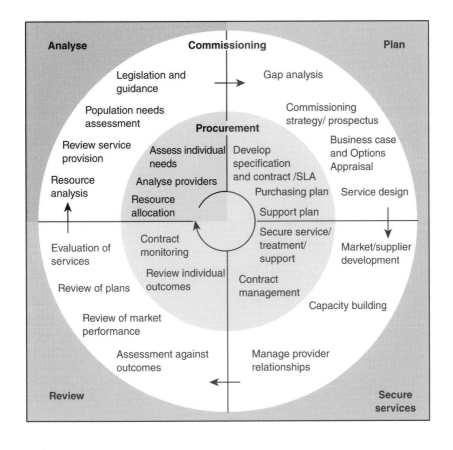

2

Why, When and How to Commission

There is nothing new under the sun. One might be forgiven for thinking sometimes, when listening to public policy pronouncements, that commissioning is a mysterious new discipline, perhaps with links to the ancient alchemists, which somehow translates tired old public services into magical shiny outcomes for service users. One might also suspect that, as with other disciplines, there is an emerging tendency by the commissioning profession to mythologise its activities and seek to protect its special expertise.

The practical reality is somewhat more prosaic. Commissioning is a series of activities which together constitute a systematic approach to planning and resourcing public services. As such, it is up to practitioners to determine how best they can organise and apply commissioning activities to help deliver better services and ultimately better outcomes for people. Everyone involved in public care, including service users and service deliverers has a role to play, activities to undertake and skills and experiences to deploy.

None of the activities involved in commissioning are new or exclusive to specialist commissioners. In many ways they are simply tasks that anyone involved in good management and practice should be doing:

- Carefully analysing a situation.
- Planning how you will deploy your resources to get the best result.
- Implementing those plans.
- Reviewing how successful you have been and deciding what needs to be done differently in future.

However, commissioning activities focus particularly on the balance of services across a market, and because of this focus, there are situations in which a systematic approach to commissioning is likely to be particularly valuable. Taking two specific examples as illustrations (older people with chronic health problems and children with special education needs), this chapter considers when and how to use commissioning and what to use it for, as well as how to ensure that the time and energy required does have a positive outcome for service users and the population as a whole.

Learning outcomes

By the end of this chapter you should be able to:

- Identify when a systematic approach to public care commissioning is and is not needed.
- Identify the most appropriate approach to commissioning for any given market.
- Plan how you would agree the purpose of a commissioning intervention with stakeholders and secure their commitment.
- Scope the kind of commissioning intervention which would be most suitable for a given situation.

When to commission?

There is a danger that, because commissioning involves many of the activities we might expect anyway from good management and professional practice, it is seen as a generic tool and it is therefore applied in almost any situation. That is not appropriate. The circumstances best suited to a commissioning approach include when:

- **There is some form of market**, i.e. a situation where those providing services need someone else to buy or to secure the services from them. This might include through contracts, service agreements, individual purchases or grants.
- **There is a need for change**, i.e. a situation where those buying or securing services want to change them to better meet the needs of service users in the future.
- **Change needs to be managed**, i.e. a situation where those involved recognise that this change needs to be undertaken deliberately and systematically and cannot simply be left to market forces.

In contrast, there are some areas where a commissioning approach is not appropriate – see Table 2.1.

Table 2.1   When a commissioning approach may not be appropriate

Commissioning is not a tool for:	Instead try:
- Internal service planning	- Business planning
- Internal re-organisation within a service	- Functional analysis - Change management
- Improving the quality of care in a particular care pathway	- Care pathway analysis and design
- Improving market position	- Market analysis and strategy

Commissioners operate at some distance from the direct management or delivery of services. They do not have the traditional 'levers' for control which exist within organisations to secure change and service improvement. They have to use different levers to secure changes in services – see Table 2.2.

Table 2.2 What levers for change may be available to commissioners

'Levers' for change available to commissioners	'Levers' for change not available to commissioners
• Influence through information and intelligence and advice to providers.	• Job descriptions.
• Influence through representation of service users and individual purchasers.	• Line management instruction.
• Influence through brokerage on behalf of service users.	• Work plans.
• Contracts with providers.	• Organisation procedures.
• Internal service level agreements with providers.	• Professional guidance.
• Market shaping through framework contracts.	• Legislation.
• Grants, gifts to encourage providers to offer particular services.	

So, commissioning is an approach to changing services across a market. It is most useful when applied to situations where the commissioning body has resources to deploy, but not day-to-day direct control over service provision. It is not the only tool for delivering services improvement but it is an important one and, when used effectively, it can secure a better deal for service users.

For example, in our two example cases, let's consider where a commissioning approach might be appropriate.

Older people with chronic health problems

- **There is some form of market**. For example a situation where health, residential and domiciliary care services are delivered by a range of providers, including the NHS, private health care providers, voluntary and private sector nursing home, care home and home care providers. In this situation there may be contracts between these providers and the local authority and NHS, as well as self-funders paying for their own care directly, and personal budget holders paying for care through direct payments from the local authority.
- **There is a need for change**. For example the commissioning bodies, primarily the NHS and local authority commissioners, have identified issues in the delivery of services for this population, including too many older people receiving poor quality care in acute services, too few services able to support people with chronic health problems in the community, and population estimates projecting a significant increase in demand over the next 10 years.

- **Change needs to be managed**. It is clear to commissioners that services are struggling to respond to demand at the current time, and that without some clear direction of travel, the market will not automatically respond by developing the most cost-effective, evidence-based services for the population.

Children with special education needs

- **There is some form of market**. For example a situation where support for parents, including respite care, school provision and residential care is provided by a range of private, voluntary and public sector providers, and commissioners contract with services from across the country to meet the individual needs of children.
- **There is a need for change**. For example the commissioning bodies, primarily the NHS and local authority commissioners, have identified that costs of services are increasing hugely, that the range of services provided do not match the needs of the population and that there are confused pathways of care and support between different services.
- **Change needs to be managed**. It is clear to commissioners that without active management of change, they will not be able to secure the services that are needed to meet the needs of their specific population of children and young people without further increases in costs.

EXERCISE 2.1

Identify a specific management or practice issue you need to address:

- Is there some form of market involved?
- Is there a need for change in services to meet the needs of a population?
- Does this change need to be managed?
- Decide, on the basis of your answers to these questions, whether you need to take a commissioning approach to the issue.

Why commission?

We all know that any public care resource is not inevitably effective. To be successful it needs to be applied in the right circumstances, efficiently, and for a clear and appropriate purpose. For example:

- A clot-busting drug is only useful when given to someone who needs it, at the right time and in the right dosage.
- A lesson on fractions is only going to be effective for a pupil with sufficient previous mathematics knowledge and the skills, resources and aptitude to learn.
- Foster care is only appropriate for a child who needs substitute care and for whom living with a family is the best available option.

Like these examples, commissioning is a particular resource, and the commissioner needs to think carefully about how and when to use it. As the later chapters in this book show, there are lots of commissioning activities which can be undertaken to help secure a successful outcome, but perhaps more important than the technical activities is that those involved are very clear about why they are using commissioning, what resources they need to apply, and what they are trying to achieve as a result.

In practice the reason behind any particular commissioning intervention will be specific to the circumstances in which it is used, but IPC has worked on many commissioning interventions for clients over the years, and has identified that there are three overall aims which they consistently try to achieve:

- To secure better outcomes for service users.
- To better match services to the needs of the population.
- To secure greater efficiency or effectiveness from services.

If you are involved in commissioning and cannot justify your activities in terms of these three aims, then you need to think again, and challenge yourself and your colleagues to clarify the purpose of the work you are doing. Returning to our two examples the following lists might comprise the main aims they are trying to achieve.

Older people with chronic health problems

The aim of the commissioning agenda for this population might be to:

- Improve the quality of care and thus the quality of life experienced by older people with chronic health problems.
- Re-distribute resources from acute to community-based care and early support.
- Ensure that new services are evidence-based and rigorously applied to secure better impact and effectiveness.

Children with special education needs

The aim of the commissioning agenda for this group of children and young people might be to:

- Improve the quality of care and education to give children a better chance of success in adulthood.
- To re-commission services so that they better meet the specific needs of individual children.

For the particular group or population you have identified, specify the aims of any commissioning intervention in terms of:

- Better outcomes for service users.
- Services better matched to the needs of the population.
- Greater efficiency or effectiveness from services.

What to commission?

Even if you are very clear that the issues you are dealing with merit a commissioning response, and that the purpose of your intervention is consistent with a commissioning agenda, you need to be realistic about your priorities and the areas that you need to focus on.

In practical terms you cannot systematically focus on changing all aspects of the public care market at the same time. You need to identify key priority areas for change and apply a realistic approach which is going to ensure you achieve your purpose using the resources that you have available. This is not something to be considered lightly. You need to make careful judgements, based on evidence, about what is needed, what is realistic, who needs to agree to the agenda, and what resources are available. Our experience is that more commissioning interventions fail because they were over-ambitious about the impact they expected to have (or unrealistic about the difficulties they were likely to encounter), rather than that they decided to address an issue which was too easy! This applies at a number of different levels:

- The overall strategic commissioning priorities for an organisation or a commissioning partnership.
- The procurement or contract management priorities.
- Individual purchasing priorities.

To make sure you are not caught out by this, there are a range of factors which you need to consider when prioritising your commissioning agenda. Ultimately you and the other key stakeholders need to take a view based on an analysis of the following:

- **Evidence from need**. A key factor in determining your commissioning priorities will be the evidence which is available about changes in future service needs or demand. So for example, clear indications from data that the number of older people with chronic health problems is going to increase, or that there will be more children with complex learning needs coming into local schools might be strong indications that a change in services is likely to be needed, and that a commissioning intervention is required.
- **Evidence from performance data**. Alternatively, there may be clear and consistent evidence from the ongoing monitoring of the activity, performance and costs of services that they

are not meeting current needs, and that changes in services are therefore required which a commissioning approach will help deliver.
- **Evidence from experience**. Finally, even if there is no immediate indication from needs or performance information that service changes are needed, there may be sufficient qualitative intelligence about gaps in service quality to indicate that issues need to be addressed strategically. This might come from sources such as service user feedback, complaints and comments, patterns in service use, or feedback over time from professionals.

However, decisions about commissioning priorities are not just technocratic in nature. The above analysis needs to be tested against the practicalities and appetite that stakeholders may have for the systematic approach to change across a market required by commissioning. This includes:

- **National policy and politics**. If it is clear that national government is encouraging public care agencies to introduce major changes in particular service areas or for particular populations, or is introducing legislation to require this, then it is likely that this will require commissioners' attention.
- **Local policy and politics**. Clear existing strategic or political commitments by local public care organisations will also drive decisions about commissioning priorities. Often partner agencies can have very different priority agendas for the same population, and it is important that joint planning bodies such as local community partnerships, health and wellbeing boards or children's partnerships have a clear role in ensuring that agendas are co-ordinated, that resources are not wasted and that providers and the public get a clear picture about areas of joint priority.
- **Local capacity**. Public agencies and their partners may, at any one time, not have sufficient resources to ensure that a systematic commissioning approach is taken to ensure the delivery of changes in services, no matter how much they are needed. It is probably a more sensible decision not to commence a commissioning project, than to waste resources in completing a half project and failing to effect any improvements.

So, what does a focused commissioning agenda actually look like? For example, in England partners within a Health and Wellbeing Board might draw on information about needs, performance and user experience, and, comparing that with local policy and priorities as well as capacity to deliver change, might agree their commissioning priorities. In our examples these might include the following.

For older people with chronic health problems

- To reduce the number of older people who require acute hospital and residential care.
- To improve the capacity of community services to support older people and their carers in their own home.
- To reduce the costs of care by encouraging services to be delivered out of hospital and delivering them locally.

For children and young people with special education needs

- To reduce the number of children who finish school with no qualifications or accredited skills.
- To encourage schools to identify children who are struggling as early as possible and address barriers to learning.
- To improve the quality of teaching and focus resources on addressing the learning needs of these children.

Each of these agendas are clearly long-term, concerned with a particular population, and are likely to require changes in systems and services across disciplines. They are commissioning agendas. They give commissioners a clear focus for their activities and, by their existence, a clear message that issues which are NOT included are not of sufficient priority to partners at the current time to warrant the level of attention that a commissioning priority will give.

As important as the priorities themselves is who has been involved in their development, and the extent to which these people are committed to supporting a commissioning intervention and possibly changing services. This is explored further in the next section, but at this analysis stage it is important to identify the key stakeholders who are likely to be affected, and begin to scope out how they will be involved in different ways in the commissioning intervention. So for example, the likely people to be involved with our two examples include:

- Local authority commissioners and planners
- NHS commissioners and planners
- Local authority providers
- NHS providers
- Existing service users
- Carers
- The public and potential future service users
- Politicians and other policy influencers
- Voluntary and private sector influencing bodies
- Professionals, clinicians and other staff involved in services

EXERCISE 2.3

For the particular group or population you have identified, name individuals and groups who need to have an influence on the commissioning intervention, and identify what level of commitment you need from them – for example, are you looking for them to offer:

- agreement with the reason changes are needed?
- contribution to the analysis?
- agreement with proposed changes?
- commitment to implementation?

Refining the agenda and getting commitment

A strategic commitment to key priorities by partner organisations is a crucial starting point for delivering change through commissioning, but it is not by any means the whole story. Such a commitment means only that it is agreed that 'something must be done' in these areas – 'what must be done' needs to be worked out. It is also always worth remembering that in most circumstances a strategic commitment by organisations to some key priorities does not mean that everyone is working on the same agenda – this commitment has not necessarily been signed up to by all of the key stakeholders such as politicians, service users and personal budget holders, professionals or all providers.

Therefore if the commissioner is an effective change agent, he or she now needs to engage with all of the key stakeholders involved, and work with them to:

- Get their input into refining the agenda and exploring the details of the issues which need to be addressed to improve services for the relevant population.
- Get their practical commitment to implementing any changes needed.

The engagement approach will need to vary here, depending upon the particular characteristics of the market, the relationship between commissioners, purchasers, service users and providers within it, and the type of influence that the commissioner is able to wield. So for example, Table 2.3 describes different market situations and how the role of the commissioner and the type of engagement required might vary.

Nevertheless, whatever the relationship between the commissioners and other key stakeholders in the market, the task of the commissioner is to facilitate change, and there are particular approaches at this stage which can be useful in drawing in stakeholders while at the same time adding depth and quality to the specification of the commissioning task.

Hypotheses

Within the boundaries of commissioning agenda, there will be some very specific priority questions that the work will need to address, to do with the issues and challenges that the stakeholders are experiencing in the market, and the emerging demands they are likely to be facing in the future. No matter what the market situation and the relationship between the commissioner and stakeholders are, introducing the opportunity to offer 'hypotheses' at this early stage of the work can help to focus minds on key issues and direct the emphasis of work onto agreed strategic commissioning priorities.

Hypotheses can be defined as 'assumptions to be used for the basis of investigation' and they can be used to enable stakeholders to identify key issues that they believe have to be explored. This ensures that key assumptions about services, however controversial, are brought out into the open. It also helps to ensure that all

Table 2.3 Market situations, the role of the commissioner and what type of engagement might be required

Market situation	Commissioner role	Engagement type
• Services funded through one large block contract (e.g. CCG contract with an acute NHS Foundation Trust)	• Commissioner is purchaser of the vast majority of services from a single independent or in-house provider on behalf of the public.	• Consultation with provider, potential providers, service users, led by commissioner. • Purpose of the consultation is to inform commissioner's future procurement and purchasing plan.
• Services purchased from a range of different contracted providers (e.g. residential or foster care provision for looked after children)	• Commissioner is purchaser of vast majority of services from a number of independent or in-house providers on behalf of the public.	• Consultation with providers, potential providers, service users led by the commissioner. • Purpose is to inform commissioner's future procurement and purchasing plans.
• Services funded through a combination of independent sources such as charities, and public contracts or grants (e.g. community-based prevention services supporting carers of older people with dementia)	• Commissioner is one of a number of funders of services who may have different priorities and plans.	• Facilitation of information sharing between different providers, potential providers, service users to establish agendas and how they might wish to engage with a strategic overview. • Purpose is to inform commissioner's future procurement and purchasing plans, and influence the behaviour of services not directly funded.
• Services purchased by personal budgets or self funders (e.g. direct payment arrangements in social care, self funders of residential care for older people, private health care)	• Commissioner is only peripherally involved in contract transactions between users and providers.	• Facilitation of information sharing between different providers, potential providers, service purchasers to establish agendas and how they might wish to engage with a strategic overview. • Purpose is to influence the behaviour of providers to meet the future needs of service users.

stakeholders have an opportunity to influence the key areas to be explored. The hypotheses also inform the details of the methodology to be used, without pre-judging the final findings.

By agreeing a selection of, say, five to eight hypotheses with key stakeholders, the agenda can be refined, and the priority issues can be agreed. So, for example, in our example of older people with chronic health problems, stakeholders might offer the hypotheses shown in Table 2.4.

Table 2.4 Older people with chronic health problems hypotheses

Population	Older people with chronic health problems
Commissioning aims	• To reduce the number of older people who require acute hospital and residential care. • To improve the capacity of community services to support older people and their carers in their own home. • To reduce the costs of care by encouraging services to be delivered out of hospital and delivering them locally.
Hypothesis 1	• Redistributing £1m currently invested in acute care for older people into community-based services will improve community support, prevent admissions and reduce demand.
Hypothesis 2	• Investing more heavily in intensive rehabilitation for older people after falls will reduce demand for residential care.
Hypothesis 3	• Redistributing £1/4m from acute sector into targeted support for carers of the most vulnerable older people will reduce demand for acute care and effect savings across the system.
Hypothesis 4	• Building more extra care housing will enable older people to live at home comfortably for longer and reduce demand for residential care.
Hypothesis 5	• Having community health and social services managed within a single organisation and working in co-terminus teams will improve efficiency and effectiveness of response, allowing more older people with chronic health problems to remain at home.
Hypothesis 6	• Many of the tasks currently undertaken by community health professionals could be undertaken by less expensive, less qualified staff, allowing us to distribute our services more widely.

Similarly, for children with special education needs, stakeholders might identify hypotheses as shown in Table 2.5.

Table 2.5 Children with special education needs hypotheses

Population	Children with Special Education Needs
Commissioning aims	• To reduce the number of children who finish school with no qualifications or accredited skills. • To encourage schools to identify children who are struggling as early as possible and address barriers to learning. • To improve the quality of teaching and focus resources on addressing the learning needs of these children.
Hypothesis 1	• Mainstream schools in the area are referring too many children to specialist resources. More children need to be better supported by these schools.
Hypothesis 2	• The 2 SEN schools in the area are not fit for purpose and need to be re-designed and re-commissioned.
Hypothesis 3	• Arrangements for identifying and sharing concerns about children who are struggling need to be improved. A common assessment framework needs to be used by all agencies.
Hypothesis 4	• Local mainstream schools need to agree a common standard and approach to teaching children with special education needs, and agree a joint training programme for teachers based on this.
Hypothesis 5	• A common protocol for support from NHS and social services staff to schools needs to be agreed.

It is crucial to ensure that these hypotheses are NOT seen by stakeholders as aims, objectives, plans or indicators – they are simply areas which need to be tested in the course of the strategic commissioning work. They can therefore be quite controversial and challenging, as long as they are concerned with issues that the stakeholders agree do need to be addressed. Subsequent work on the strategic commissioning intervention will need to test these hypotheses out, and come to a view about whether they should be translated into commissioning aims or objectives.

EXERCISE 2.4

• For your chosen population prepare a series of hypotheses that you want to test out in the course of the commissioning intervention.
• Make sure they are phrased in the form of statements, and for each, identify how you might collect information which would allow you to test the hypothesis.

Commissioning jointly

At the same time as building hypotheses together, it is important that partners are able to commit themselves to the results of any strategic commissioning initiative, and, wherever possible to undertake commissioning activities together. Where there is a common agreed agenda this can have the following benefits:

- All services relevant to the wellbeing of the population concerned can be considered – such as, for children with special education needs, the range of health, education and social care provision.
- Commissioning resources can be shared.
- Budgets can be pooled.

Joint commissioning in practice, however, means many different things to different people, and it is important for partners to be clear about the approach they are taking to commissioning together right from the start of any intervention. IPC has found that approaches can be summarised under four headings, as shown in Table 2.6.

Table 2.6 The four commissioning approaches

Separate approaches	Parallel approaches
Objectives, plans, actions and decisions are arrived at independently and without co-ordination.	Objectives, plans, actions and decisions are arrived at with reference to other agencies.
Joint approaches	**Integrated approaches**
Objectives, plans, actions and decisions are developed in partnership by separate agencies.	Objectives, plans, actions and decisions are arrived at through a single organisation or network.

Despite the enthusiasm from national policy-makers across the UK for integrated health and social care, we have found that integrated approaches to commissioning are not inevitably better. It depends upon the situation that the partners are dealing with and there may be different types of activity depending upon the specific commissioning intervention that partners are undertaking. So for example, in our case study examples, partners might agree the following:

- For older people with chronic health problems – to adopt an integrated approach to health and social care commissioning including pooled budgets, as the health and social care needs of the population involved are so closely entwined.
- For children and young people with special educational needs – to adopt a parallel approach to commissioning between education and social care services, as local budgets held by schools would be difficult to aggregate up to pool with social care.

In the appendix to this chapter the IPC joint commissioning matrix describes some of the different approaches in more detail.

EXERCISE 2.5

- Use the IPC joint commissioning matrix to discuss the approach you need to take to joint commissioning with your partners.

Formalising the commitment of different partners

Negotiating the arrangements described in the sections above is often tricky, needing a degree of patience and good understanding of the different perspectives of the range of stakeholders involved in the whole commissioning process, and finding ways to ensure that all are clear about the overall task and about their involvement and responsibilities. One way of securing this commitment is to agree and publish a 'Commissioning Framework', a document which summarises these commitments and provides a realistic and sensible guide about how commissioning activities are expected to be undertaken. The framework might include:

- Definitions of commissioning, planning, procurement and associated terms.
- Principles which underpin the local approach to commissioning.
- A summary of the activities undertaken within the commissioning process.
- Who does what including organisations, teams and individuals.
- A list of key documents published by partners and how they relate to each other.
- How different partners, including service users, carers, the public and providers can expect to be involved in commissioning decisions.
- Legislation and policy which underpin the approach to commissioning by different partners.
- A programme and timetable of activities throughout the year relevant to partners.

Its value is primarily in ensuring that partners think through potential problems and difficulties beforehand, and have a resource to help them resolve problems as they work together.

EXERCISE 2.6

- Review the existing policy and guidance documents in your local area, and decide whether they are clear about the approach which is used to underpin commissioning practice locally. If they are not, work with partners to design and publish a commissioning framework.

Designing the strategic commissioning intervention

Deciding what form of commissioning interventions are needed in a particular situation needs careful judgement and needs to be based upon:

- A clear idea of the purpose of the intervention and what you hope to achieve.
- A detailed understanding of the market involved, the interests of different stakeholders and what you need to work on to achieve change.
- A good analysis of what different activities can offer and when they are likely to be most effective.

Obviously all of the activities within the IPC commissioning framework (described in Chapter 1) are commissioning interventions, but in this section of four of the most common types of intervention are summarised, along with the circumstances under which they might prove most useful.

After the outline in this chapter, the activities involved are discussed in more detail throughout the rest of the book.

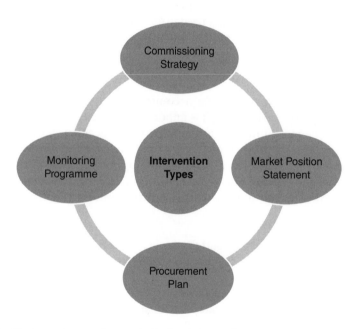

Figure 2.1   Common types of commissioning intervention

A commissioning strategy

The key characteristic of a commissioning strategy is that it presents an authoritative analysis of current arrangements and future needs for a given population, and states clearly where the commissioners intend to spend their money.

Producing commissioning strategies involves undertaking research and analysis activities to produce a document which has been agreed formally by the commissioning organisations involved and includes:

- A statement about how the strategy has been developed, and who has been involved.
- An overview of how the strategy addresses the outcomes and intended aims of the agencies involved and other commitments such as national policy and legislation for the relevant population group.
- An overview of national guidance and research relevant to the specific group being considered.
- An assessment of the health, education, social care and other needs of the relevant population taking into account user and staff views.
- An analysis of the extent and effectiveness of current resources, and potential service improvements.
- An analysis of gaps and overlaps in services, and priorities for where services need to be redeveloped, reduced or increased.
- A plan for the pattern of services to be purchased in the future, including where resources will be targeted and where there may need to be service de-commissioning.
- A statement about arrangements for future procurement, contracting and market management.
- A statement about how the strategy will be monitored and reviewed.

The activities involved in developing a commissioning strategy are described in detail in later chapters. At this point it is important to be clear about why and where a strategy might be most appropriate, so that you can decide whether or not to put time and energy into its production. As we have discussed, a strategy needs to be based on the starting point for all commissioning interventions – some form of market – a need for change; and that change requiring to be managed. However, there are particular circumstances which lend themselves to a strategy including where:

- Commissioners have a very large part to play in purchasing services within the market, and have a key influence over the resources which go into services for the population concerned.
- Commissioners need to be public about where they are going to focus their resources, and about how they plan to focus their procurement and purchasing in future.

A market position statement

A market position statement (MPS) has many of the characteristics (described in detail in Chapter 8) and involves many of the same activities as a commissioning strategy but is different in some fundamental ways:

- It is an analytical, 'market facing' document that brings together material from sources such as strategic plans and commissioning strategies into a document that presents the data that providers within the market need to know if they are to plan their future role and function.

- It signals the commissioners' desired model of practice for a specific market segment, and how they will seek to influence providers who are not funded directly to provide those services.
- Indicates the necessary changes, characteristics and innovation to service design and delivery the commissioner identifies as needed to meet the needs and preferences of the population using those services, and how commissioners will support and intervene in those markets.

It is this analytical element – and its focus on information that providers need to know to develop their own businesses and service – which characterises the MPS in comparison with a commissioning strategy. An MPS might for example, have the elements shown in Table 2.7.

Table 2.7 Elements of a Market Position Statement

- A summary of the direction the commissioning organisation(s) wish to take and the purpose of the document
- The commissioning organisation's(s') predictions of future demand, identifying key pressure points
- The commissioning organisation's(s') picture of the current state of supply covering both strengths and weaknesses within the market
- Identified models of practice the commissioning organisation(s) will encourage
- The likely future level of resourcing
- The support the commissioning organisation(s) will offer towards providing choice as well as innovation and development

An MPS is particularly useful in the following market contexts:

- Where the commissioners are not the primary contract holders. This is an increasingly common situation in England for example:

  o Where individual adults requiring social care or families of children with disabilities are given direct payments or personal budgets with which to purchase their own care. This means that the local authority (unless asked) which previously purchased services on behalf of these populations is no longer involved in the choice of provider or the detailed contracting of services. In effect resources have been handed over to the individual service user to contract and manage.
  o Where individuals are funding the purchase of care for themselves because they are too wealthy to qualify for state support.
  o Where individual schools are managing their own budgets and purchasing support services rather than using the local authority to provide them.

- Where changes in the market need to be influenced or managed. In the situations described above, one might argue that the market could be left to itself to regulate and to balance, but most sectors and commentators agree that local commissioners have an important role to play in market facilitation – or ensuring that information about activity, need, quality and availability is available and that vital services are not allowed to fail. An MPS can help with this.

- Where information about services to inform choice is not easily available. Many of the services provided via the public care sector are highly regulated, complicated, and the subject of a purchasing decision by members of the public on only very rare occasions. The role of the commissioner is to make sure the information available is accessible and of good quality to help purchasers make good decisions and an MPS is an important tool to help this.

A procurement exercise

Procurement is the process of acquiring goods and services, and, where the commissioner is also a holder of funds, is a key stage in securing local services to meet needs efficiently and effectively. Procurement activities do need to be driven by the intelligence and analysis gathered in a commissioning strategy, and they can involve the following:

- Tendering for contracted services from third sector or private providers.
- Developing service-level agreements with providers operating from within the public sector.
- Providing grants to voluntary organisations to help them deliver services.
- Setting framework contracts with providers which specify the services and rates which will be charged to individuals if and when they spot purchase from them in future.

Procurement activities in the public sector are subject to national and European legislation and guidance designed to ensure that opportunities are made available fairly and that the public sector gets good value for money. These are considered further in a later chapter. At this point it is worth noting that a procurement exercise is a commissioning intervention particularly worth considering when:

- A commissioner has resources which it needs to use cost-effectively to secure best outcomes for service users.
- The strategic intentions of the commissioner in a market are clear, and based on good evidence and detailed analysis.
- There is good data and analysis about the quality and performance of existing services.

A monitoring programme

The final major commissioning intervention is related to all of the previous three examples, but is included as a separate type of intervention because of the frequency with which commissioners come to recognise that they need to commence with monitoring of existing services before embarking on one of the other interventions.

A monitoring intervention is essentially an opportunity for a commissioner to set up systems which enable them to get a good grasp of the characteristics of the local market. It is not about undertaking a one-off exercise, but rather setting up arrangements which will enable commissioners to be better informed on an ongoing basis. For example, it might involve setting up arrangements for:

- Monitoring changes in population growth and demand on services.
- Reviewing the performance of services through monitoring progress in national inspections.
- Reviewing the impact of services by reviewing the outcomes achieved by service users.
- Reviewing the performance and quality of services through monitoring user and carer feedback.
- Monitoring performance against contract in terms of activities undertaken, services providers, users supported, costs incurred and outcomes achieved.

This information is crucial if commissioners are to work effectively with service providers and if they are to be able to facilitate markets with skill and insight. However, it is difficult to collect on a consistent basis and requires considerable time and commitment. Circumstances in which such interventions are most appropriate include:

- Where commissioners recognise the value of good quality market information and are willing to invest in securing it.
- Where commissioners are either major service purchasers, or where they are able to agree with providers that there is a market facilitation role which needs to be informed by good quality ongoing service and quality data.

Case studies

Going back to our case studies, we have already established the need for a commissioning intervention in both situations; we have identified the aims of the interventions and some key hypotheses which need to be addressed by the intervention. We have also identified key stakeholders and how they might be engaged in any intervention. Finally, drawing on the sections above, we need to propose the most appropriate type of intervention.

Older people with chronic health problems

In this case, we might agree that the primary change is likely to be a shift in resources from acute to community services, and that this will involve re-commissioning of NHS resources. Therefore we might decide that joint commissioning partners will use the development of a commissioning strategy to make the case for this re-distribution, identify the changes required and to specify which key contracts will need to be re-negotiated.

Children with special education needs

In this situation, with the local authority working with a range of independent budget holding schools, it might be impractical to develop a commissioning strategy covering all of the intentions of the commissioners, so the local authority might work on a market position statement to give an indication to service providers about the market as a whole and how it is likely to develop.

- Consider again the population you have been looking at throughout this chapter. Which of the four major commissioning interventions do you need to consider for this population at the current time?
- Why is this approach the right one for the circumstances?

Summary

This chapter has been concerned with the whys, the whens and the hows of commissioning. By now, if you have considered the examples and completed all of the exercises you should have a pretty clear idea about your own commissioning priorities, who you need to engage with to develop your commissioning intervention, and what kind of commissioning activities you need to undertake.

Commissioning is about change in organisations, in services and most fundamentally in people. As such it will always involve compromise, contingencies and careful judgement, and guidelines such as those in this chapter will not replace the local knowledge you need to apply in practice. However, a clear rationale, a good route map and a clear destination can help to ensure that the purpose of a commissioning intervention is not lost in the middle of the day-to-day work on improving public care.

Further reading and web-based resources

There are a number of web-based resources which explore these issues in more detail and provide up-to-date resources including:

Commissioning Support Programme Developed for the Department for Education originally, it covers resources to support children's commissioning. Available at: www. commissioningsupport.org.uk/

Intelligent Commissioning. Developed by IPC for the Yorkshire and The Humber Region, it covers resources for commissioning adult social care services. Available at: www.yhsccommissioning.org.uk

Buy4Wales Commissioning Route Planner Based on the IPC commissioning framework this website provides extensive guidance and resources to inform social care commissioning and procurement particularly but not exclusively in Wales. It also gives access to the national commissioning framework and guidance produced by the Welsh Assembly in 2010, which uses the IPC framework as its basis. Available at: www.buy4wales.co.uk/PRP/social-care

Joint Improvement Team Scotland Commissioning Guidance This guidance, based on the IPC commissioning framework covers good joint commissioning practice for partner agencies across Scotland. Available at: www.jitscotland.org.uk/action-areas/commissioning/

Appendix

Joint commissioning tool – a matrix for analysing approaches to commissioning across agencies

IPC has drawn on a range of materials and its own experience of working on the commissioning of public care services throughout the country to develop a matrix for analysing the extent to which different areas of the commissioning and contracting process are integrated across agencies. The matrix uses the following seven commissioning and contracting areas:

- Purpose and strategy
- Needs and market intelligence
- Stakeholder engagement
- Resource allocation and management
- Market management and monitoring
- Contracting
- Commissioning function

The matrix also differentiates between the following four levels of integration:

- Separate approaches: Actions and decisions are arrived at independently and without co-ordination.
- Parallel approaches: Objectives, plans, actions and decisions are arrived at with reference to other agencies.
- Joint approaches: Objectives, plans, actions and decisions are developed in partnership by separate agencies.
- Integrated approaches: Objectives, plans, actions and decisions are arrived at through a single organisation or network.

Examples of activities at each level are described in Figure 2.2 below.

Areas	Separate approaches	Parallel approaches	Joint approaches	Integrated approaches
Purpose and strategy	• Agencies develop services to meet their own priorities. • Single agency planning documents do not include key partners' priorities and drivers. • Single-agency commissioning strategies.	• Systematic analysis of partner agency perspectives, issues and concerns. • Liaison in the production of separate strategies. • Strategies reference and address partners' issues.	• Shared commitment to improve outcomes across client group. • Joint strategy development teams producing common strategies.	• Inclusive planning and decision process as an integral partner. • A transparent relationship between integrated bodies. • Single agency with one commissioning function.
Needs and market intelligence	• Needs analysis is undertaken independently, and deals with very specific aspects of population need. • Agencies use provider intelligence for the purpose of identifying their own commissioning priorities only.	• Separate needs analyses shared by agencies. • Separate cost, benchmarking and general market intelligence shared by agencies.	• Jointly designed population needs analysis. • Joint working groups to review market mix.	• Single projects undertaking needs and market analysis and using these to inform commissioning and contracting priorities. • Single research, analysis, public health teams.
Stakeholder engagement	• Public meetings, conferences, feedback are designed and delivered independently.	• Information from service users or service providers is shared when clearly relevant.	• Agencies jointly design and manage consultation and feedback activities.	• A single team is responsible for systematic planning and delivery of provider consultation to inform a single strategy.

Areas	Separate approaches	Parallel approaches	Joint approaches	Integrated approaches
Resource allocation and management	• Budgets are used solely to meet self-determined objectives. • The financial impact of services and policies on other agencies is not considered.	• Agencies allocate some resources to address issues of common concern.	• Agencies identify pooled budgets for particular areas, and a joint approach to decision making on budget allocation to meet common objectives. • Use of Health Act Flexibilities.	• Pooled budgets within a single agency or network, to meet combined needs identified for the population.
Market management and monitoring	• Market management sited in separate organisations. • A fragmented approach to use of providers and resources. • Provider performance information not shared between agencies.	• Performance measurement information shared to promote commonality and consistency. • Agencies inform each other of performance improvement needs.	• Multi-agency review groups ensure robust joint arrangements for the collection and interpretation of performance information. • Sharing of risk with market development	• Integrated monitoring and review arrangements that result in a shared understanding of the effectiveness of current services and the evidence for changes in the future.
Contracting	• Contract compliance information is used independent of other sources and solely within the organisation.	• Agencies inform each other of purchasing intentions. • Agencies share information about contracts and intelligence about performance where relevant.	• Agencies issue joint block contracts or share contract risk. • Standard joint contract terms are realistic and deliverable by providers.	• Single function responsible for managing contracts to meet a single commissioning agenda.

(Continued)

Figure 2.2   (Continued)

Areas	Separate approaches	Parallel approaches	Joint approaches	Integrated approaches
Commissioning functions	• Agencies have their own teams to support their commissioning activities.	• Agencies liaise re commissioning activities (e.g. needs analysis, monitoring of individual agency strategies) in order to support common commissioning objectives. • Identified common training and development needs within agencies.	• Emerging hybrid roles support a joint strategic commissioning function across agencies. • A clear understanding of the resources and skills required to provide support to joint strategic commissioning. • Joint appointments of commissioning staff.	• Integrated commissioning function, e.g. a single manager with responsibility for managing commissioning and contracting within a single organisation or network.

Figure 2.2   Joint commissioning matrix

3

Conducting Strategic Needs Assessments

Understanding data through a needs analysis is essential to inform and review commissioning decisions; the foundation of the commissioning process is a picture of the population, its local communities and their public care needs. It is important for commissioners to understand the needs and aspirations of whole populations and how these are influenced by the varying needs of individuals.

Ideally, as part of the commissioning process, information on needs should be combined with data on research, legislation and national guidance as well as reviewing current provision in terms of the range, quality and costs of services. Commissioners' understanding of need can then be compared to information about what services are being provided (see Chapter 4 on mapping services) to assess whether money is being spent wisely.

A needs analysis is a way of estimating the nature and extent of the needs of a population so that services can be planned accordingly. Strategic needs analyses cover populations and can be segmented for example by ethnicity, gender, disability, looked after status, risk of criminality, geographical location. They can be for the immediate future or long term. 'Strategic' means it is concerned with population rather than individual needs, although much aggregation of data from such sources can contribute at a strategic level.

Learning outcomes

By the end of this chapter you should be able to:

- Understand why strategic needs assessments are needed as the platform for change.
- Understand what resources are required to achieve optimum results.
- Analyse the needs of or demand for services from the population.
- Create evidence-based strategic needs assessments.

Key terms

- *Needs* – a judgement that individuals or groups lack something (income, education, housing, or social care for example) that they ought to have, or that they have fallen below some minimum level
- *Demands* – users' or patients' wants or requests for service or support
- *Supply or resource analysis* – an analysis looking at the resources or supply of services available to meet need in a given area or market
- *Market intelligence* – a common and shared perspective of supply and demand, leading to an evidenced, published, market position statement for a given market
- *Strategic needs assessments (SNAs)* – in our context any assessments that identify 'the big picture', in terms of the health and wellbeing needs and inequalities of a local population. Joint strategic needs assessments (JSNAs) are one step further and are a mandatory requirement for health and social care agencies designed to help organisations with service planning and the commissioning process. SNAs and JSNAs are used interchangeably in the text.

Why is it important to have an evidenced-based strategic needs assessment?

In essence you cannot commission cost-effective services that deliver good outcomes unless you know the purpose of the commissioning in terms of needs that will be met through the process; this is one of the key roles of a commissioner. The reasons often given to support this statement are that SNAs allow commissioners to:

- Select the best interventions and services.
- Ensure that there is a range and capacity of services available and accessible.
- Enable the more effective and economic configuration of services.
- Provide a clearer idea of what is needed and at what cost.
- Deliver what people want and improve the personal experience of services.
- Performance manage and incentivise providers.
- Evidence decisions to enable stakeholders to buy-in to change.

Further, the assessment process as a whole ensures services can be mapped to outcomes or resources. It can highlight where there are overlaps and gaps which in turn help to show which services should be commissioned, commissioned differently or decommissioned. If the SNA includes a spend analysis for the authority or agency it will also contain key financial information for service planning and performance such as overall spend on services, key spend areas, number of providers having contracts and their service profiles.

Joint strategic needs assessments (JSNAs)

Integrated health and social care is still seen by many as vital for better outcomes for service users and patients while making limited resources go further (Humphries and Curry, 2011). The format that public services use in England to undertake such needs assessments will be that of a joint strategic needs assessment which came into being with the Local Government and Public Involvement in Health Act 2007.

A JSNA is the means by which local NHS commissioners and local authorities jointly describe the future health, care and wellbeing needs of local populations and the strategic direction of service delivery to meet those needs. The focus of a JSNA should be on outcomes, partnership working and consultation and it should drive the commissioning process. Very often, however, this does not occur and JSNAs can become, like many large scale studies of need, mere volumes of data unused by commissioners.

A recent national review looked in depth at a sample of JSNAs and found a range of issues (IPC, 2010: 3):

- All JSNAs reflected broad concerns about the health and wellbeing of the communities they covered.
- JSNAs varied widely in terms of length, focus and content.
- Although in some instances there had been a written agreement over what the JSNA was to focus on, in others there was not, which when linked to the absence of strategic commissioners from 'setting up' discussions was probably crucial in understanding why the JSNA did not focus more on key commissioning decisions.
- In some instances there was a tendency to present snapshot, rather than trend, data. The latter would have provided a better basis from which future predictions could have been made.
- Providers were rarely involved in giving demand information from the perspective of the services they provided, although they were more likely to be involved in discussions on the finished document.
- There appeared to be little involvement of housing strategy managers as commissioners in the development of the JSNA. The same would be true of planners.
- Some topic areas such as learning disability did not offer a detailed analysis of future predictions of demand.
- Some commissioning strategies contained detailed information about demand that was not derived from the JSNA.
- In general JSNAs did not review and analyse data about supply.

Although this study did not claim to be fully representative, it does appear that these issues remain commonplace.

The process of developing a strategic needs assessment

Figure 3.1 gives an overview of the process of constructing a SNA moving from the agreement of its specification and collecting data, through to implementation and reviewing the value of the whole process.

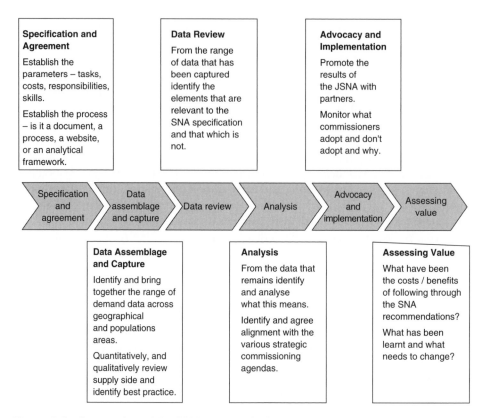

Specification and Agreement

Establish the parameters – tasks, costs, responsibilities, skills.

Establish the process – is it a document, a process, a website, or an analytical framework.

Data Review

From the range of data that has been captured identify the elements that are relevant to the SNA specification and that which is not.

Advocacy and Implementation

Promote the results of the JSNA with partners.

Monitor what commissioners adopt and don't adopt and why.

Specification and agreement › Data assemblage and capture › Data review › Analysis › Advocacy and implementation › Assessing value

Data Assemblage and Capture

Identify and bring together the range of demand data across geographical and populations areas.

Quantitatively, and qualitatively review supply side and identify best practice.

Analysis

From the data that remains identify and analyse what this means.

Identify and agree alignment with the various strategic commissioning agendas.

Assessing Value

What have been the costs / benefits of following through the SNA recommendations?

What has been learnt and what needs to change?

Figure 3.1 An overview of the SNA process (IPC, 2010)

Worthy of particular consideration is the key decision regarding the initial specification for the SNA. This is about choosing between a broad-based view of health and wellbeing from which future health and social care commissioning priorities should be derived i.e. breadth *or*, a focus on the key commissioning decisions that have to be made and how the SNA can help commissioners to make those judgements (depth). The choice is illustrated in Figure 3.2.

One argument could of course be that the SNA needs to do both. However, even if it is considered that the two are compatible, in resource terms there may simply not be the capacity to offer a broad-based view at the same time as drilling down into data in order to understand the detail behind demand and how it may be addressed. Commissioners and analysts will need to strike the balance between this broad view and drilling down in a way that meets local requirements.

If the SNA is to play an important role in strategic commissioning then its own procurement needs to be undertaken in a structured way. There should be discussion and debate, but there also needs to be a process around which a clear written agreement can be constructed and a value ascribed to the SNA activity. The following should be covered by such an agreement:

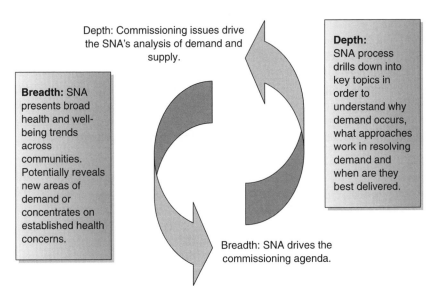

Depth: Commissioning issues drive the SNA's analysis of demand and supply.

Depth:
SNA process drills down into key topics in order to understand why demand occurs, what approaches work in resolving demand and when are they best delivered.

Breadth: SNA presents broad health and well-being trends across communities. Potentially reveals new areas of demand or concentrates on established health concerns.

Breadth: SNA drives the commissioning agenda.

Figure 3.2   Depth v. breadth as the focus for the SNA

- Determining the extent and focus: If local government, health care and other commissioners need analytical information from the SNA which can be used to target provision, then there is a need to specify the issues and resource decisions that may be required. This may cover information about demand and supply, an understanding of where that data is currently located and the hypotheses the analysis would seek to test. In the case of falls, for example, it may be that current falls provision is not targeted enough on the right populations with proven methodologies to have maximum possible impact for the minimum acceptable price.
- Understanding commissioning decisions: To deliver the above is likely to require SNA authors to have a clear idea about the commissioning context and areas of demand to be targeted and why. What kind of analysis is required to fit the demands of the commissioning strategy?
- Partners: There needs to be clarity at the outset about who is to be involved – as an author; as a contributor of data; as a customer of the information and analysis that the SNA offers. It was mentioned earlier that partners such as strategic housing appeared to play little part in both the development of the SNAs and in receiving information as a potential customer. Yet for example, data and analysis from Strategic Housing Market Assessments could make a useful contribution to the analysis. Similarly, provider services have considerable repositories of data about service users and large organisations have a keen understanding of the market, which it may be beneficial for the SNA to incorporate.
- Process and product: The implicit assumption from the original government guidance was of the SNA being a single written document. However, this may not represent the best use of time and resources. Some authorities are already producing subject specific SNAs relating to particular aspects of need, e.g. mental health, older people etc. In some areas there are discussions about 'augmenting the Index of Multiple Deprivation and the SNA with a "joint strategic assets assessment"' (Foot and Hopkins, 2010). There may be a need to take all this much further and see the SNA authors as a standing group of advisors on demand and

supply that is available to partners to call on. Figure 3.3 illustrates the relationship between breadth and depth and process versus product in defining what type of SNA is produced.

- Logistics and resources: If the role of the SNA is extended there are clearly resource implications that will need to be dealt with at the specification stage. Resource considerations may also involve reviewing data availability. If the end product is to be a written product it is clear from the review that there is scope for reducing the level of description and upping the analytical content. For commissioners the question may not be 'what data is available?' but, 'how do I draw conclusions from the information that I am being presented with?'

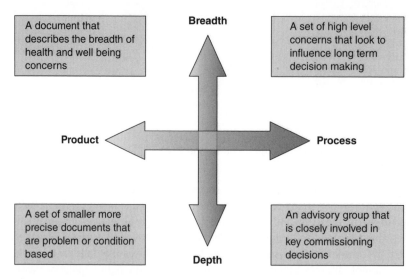

Figure 3.3   Balancing the output of the SNA with its focus

Stop and Reflect

Take a moment to stop and reflect on your own organisation and its current SNA process.

- Is there a clear specification for SNA authors?
- Is the balance between a broad view and drilling down struck in a way that meets local need?
- Is there engagement by all parts of the community in the SNA commissioning process and are they active recipients of its products?
- Should the SNA become more than a document and instead provide a permanent analytical resource for decision making at the health, housing and social care and wider public service interface?
- Is the local SNA community fully engaged with the concept of an asset approach to reducing inequalities and considering the balance between this and deficit-based approaches?
- Would the current specification be adequate to meet the requirements of CCGs?

Needs and supply analyses

Although social and health 'demand' for resources is not identical conceptually to 'need', they are clearly linked (see the definitions above). To support effective commissioning an SNA should therefore include information on demand. In addition, the best SNAs need to supplement a 'pure' SNA with a supply or resource analysis. This section therefore looks at these two interrelated elements of need/demand and resource analyses in turn and how they link together. The resource mapping aspect of assessment activity is examined in more detail in Chapter 5.

Need and demand analysis

Following the Health and Social Care Act 2011 JSNAs have had a more pointed brief (NHS Confederation, 2011):

> The outcome, or product, of a JSNA process can include different ways of organising or presenting data, such as online resources, thematic maps or tables. The JSNA should reflect the needs of a local population, not just the demand for services, although this too may be important to consider. Data quality is important to ensure assessments accurately reflect the needs of a population. Clinical commissioning groups (CCGs) and local authorities will be free to choose JSNA products that offer the most value and best meet the needs of target audiences.

For health, social care and other agencies the JSNA (or products from it) should contain analyses of the following:

- Population level demography: age, gender, ethnicity, population growth and migration flows including estimates of future demands, e.g. a profile of the local current baseline population and projections of how that population is likely to change over time. This will allow commissioners to understand the characteristics of their population.
- Wider population future demands: needs, expectations and desires are changing – it is important to try and understand how this will affect future demand.
- Social, economic and environmental determinants of health: housing quality, environment, employment, educational attainment, benefit uptake, crime, community cohesion, and community assets such as libraries.
- Behavioural determinants of health and consequent care demands: exercise, smoking, diet, alcohol and drug use, immunisation uptake, domestic violence.
- Epidemiology: incidence and prevalence of physical and mental illness and wellbeing, quality of life, life expectancy. This includes prevalence and incidence data to estimate the size of the target populations, their demographic profiles and the type and severity of need.
- Local data collected by public bodies and providers around service access and use: residential and day care, self-funders, emergency hospital admissions, nursing home admissions, health and community provider services and data, discharge information, and children's centres.
- National research findings and evidence of effectiveness: good practice examples, reviews of academic evidence, NICE guidelines and quality standards.

- Community, patient and service user perspectives: views, perceptions and experiences of patients, service users and local communities; and their physical, emotional, social and physiological needs. This includes detailed information on people who use services where there is likely to be the use of qualitative methods to gather data – perhaps focus groups and questionnaires. This will also include consultation results/press articles/perception data.
- Risk factor data: for example, to identify the likelihood of children and young people requiring services.

Figure 3.4 from the Care Services Efficiency Delivery (CSED) programme summarises how these data can be organised as a demand analysis in four stages showing existing needs, expressed demand, service take-up and lastly gaps around unmet need and outcomes.

More will be said about the tools and methodologies to achieve this type of analysis later in Chapter 6.

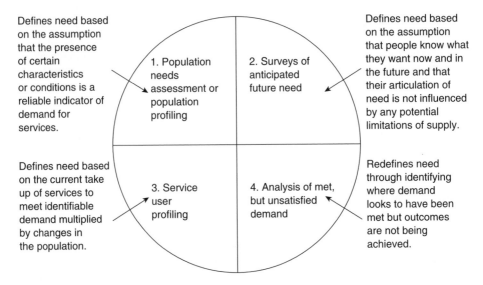

Figure 3.4 Mapping demand (CSED, 2007)

Supply analysis

Following the needs analysis, it is crucial to have an understanding of the resources available in order to help identify commissioning priorities and decision making. This is often the time that specific related market intelligence activities can be initiated such as formulating market position statements (see Chapter 8)

Resource, service or supply analysis is where the focus then turns to understand what is currently available, and what might be available in the future to meet needs. This analysis needs ultimately to allow the commissioners to make key judgements such as:

- Whether services are well aligned with the needs of the population.
- Whether the quality of services is good enough.
- Whether services present good value for money.
- Whether there are significant risks of service failure or deterioration.

To allow these judgements to be made, information is required which will answer some key questions such as:

- What services are currently provided?
- What organisations – and with what constitution, governance and resources – provide them?
- How are they differentiated – for instance geographically, by user group, gender or age?
- What are the volumes of activity, cost and quality of these services?
- What type of contract arrangements exist for these services?
- What budgets and finances are available for services, now and in the future?
- What changes to provision could existing providers offer, and who are other potential providers of these services?
- What do service users and carers say about the quality of services?
- What do recent inspections say about the quality of services?

To gather this information needs patience and resourcefulness involving, usually, a combination of activities including:

- Written questionnaires to existing and potential service providers to gather basic information.
- Review of spot, block and cost/volume contracts, Service Level Agreements (SLAs) and grants from the local authority and the Clinical Commissioning Groups.
- Mapping services by factors such as geographical area, level of need, gender, race or age.
- A detailed analysis of the experience of a small sample of service users by tracking their journeys through the care pathway between different services, to identify the extent to which services have been successful in meeting their needs.
- Finance and budget analysis and projection.
- Interviews and focus groups with service users and carers.

The importance and sometimes lack of attention to resource analysis is well expressed in the following extract from a study of commissioning strategies (Moultrie, 2007):

In contrast to the need analysis stage, the danger is rarely that too much information is collected here – more frequently the problem is that the information is not available, patchy, unreliable, old or difficult to compare between one service and another. Unless you are dealing with a very limited market situation (such as, for example, where all services for the population are provided by a single provider) it is at this stage where most energy and effort needs to be focused. The credibility of the commissioner depends heavily on having an understanding of the entire market – something that no other stakeholder is able to offer, and collecting this information together is a key indication of this credibility.

Figure 3.5 gives a diagrammatic picture of the mapping of supply which underlies the resource analysis. This CSED Programme model, as in the approach to demand, focuses on four stages of data analysis which takes into account both quantitative and qualitative data about provider services in addition to costs, best value and quality.

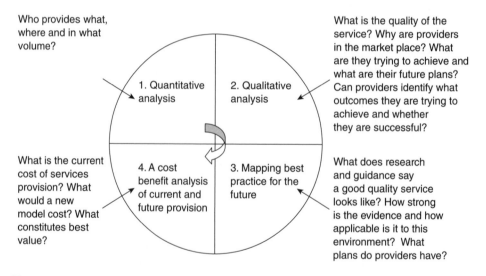

Figure 3.5 Mapping supply (CSED, 2007)

Having undertaken both the need and resource analyses of an SNA, commissioners are then in a good position to carry out other important activities, such as:

- Doing a gap analysis between demand and supply.
- Drawing conclusions about earlier commissioning or service 'hypotheses'.
- Making service design proposals for consultation.
- Producing a market position statement.
- Formulating commissioning strategies.

Methodologies and data sources

An SNA is a way of estimating the nature and extent of the needs of a population so that services can be planned and the section above has listed some of the information that service planners and commissioners will want to know about need and services (demand and supply). Typically data will need to be interrogated to see if it can help with a range of questions, for example:

- What current services are available?
- What is the profile of service users?
- How much does the service cost in total and per head?
- What are service users' and carers' views of the service?
- Does the service provide good value for money?
- Who is not getting this service that might need it?
- What is future demand likely to be?
- How could the service be improved?
- Are there other, more effective ways to deliver the outcomes which this service aims to address?
- What is the impact of the service on the overall system?

To help answer these questions the SNA needs to use a range of methodologies to gather the data appropriately and help turn them into useful information.

Qualitative vs. quantitative

Typically both qualitative and quantitative data/methods need to be used together as indicated in the CSED models above. These two different methodologies can generally be distinguished according to what they are best used for.

- Quantitative – good for answering questions of how many, how much, how long. Example uses are: in systematic reviews; randomised controlled trials; quasi-experimental studies; pre-post studies
- Qualitative – good for looking at meanings, experiences and views. Example uses are: interviews; focus groups; observational studies; visual and creative methods

Figure 3.6 gives more detail of the different characteristics of the two approaches with some illustrations.

In terms of identifying and collecting the data for an SNA, a realistic balance needs to be struck between quantitative and qualitative sources. An appropriate combination of sources might be:

- National and international research as well as government guidance and legislation.
- Population data and prevalence rates.

- Referral, assessment and service activity data.
- Illustrative care pathway/case studies.
- Engagement activities with patients/service users and carers, providers, professionals and other stakeholders.

	Quantitative *How many? How much? How long?*	Qualitative *Meanings, experiences and views*
AIM	Forecast; estimate; measurement.	Understanding processes; explanation; generation of ideas.
EMPHASIS	Breadth of understanding; extensive coverage.	In-depth and detailed; intensive coverage.
SCALE	Minimum detail from maximum number of cases.	Maximum detail from minimum number of cases.
SAMPLE	Larger sample sizes; numerically representative.	Small sample; typically researcher selects sample.
USEFUL FOR…	Description of patterns or trends; measurement of extent, location or differences.	Exploratory work where issues are not clearly understood; complex or sensitive issues.
ANALYSIS	Reduces what people say to a number of standard categories.	Enables the experiences and dialogue of the people being studied to be observed.
OUTPUT	Numerical testing of hypotheses; can make (statistical) generalisations about the wider population based on the findings drawn from a sample of individuals.	Can make generalisations about the meaning of relationships and events; represents what we looking at in a non-statistical way.
FOR EXAMPLE	What are the characteristics of men who attend family centre programmes? How do the health and well-being scores of adults with learning disabilities in residential accommodation differ from those of adults with learning disabilities living in housing in the community? What is the impact on educational attainment of looked-after young people who do not attend their reviews? Will paying supplements to foster carers that are contingent upon examination success improve the academic performance of fostered children? What is the most effective way to prevent repeated episodes of self-harm?	Why are many men reluctant to attend programmes at family centres? What is the range of opinions held by adults with learning disabilities about the respective merits of residential accommodation and housing in the community? Why do some looked-after young people prefer not to attend their reviews? What are the views of fostered children on educational incentive payments to foster carers? Why do some young people self-harm?

Figure 3.6 Characteristics and use of quantitative and qualitative research methods (Cabinet Office, 2008) Available at: www.commissioningsupport.org.uk/idoc219b. pdf?docid=b3d8a6fe-3d39-4962-ac07-d4932b57f&version=-1

www.civilservice.gov.uk/wp-content/uploads/2011/09/a_quality_framework_tcm6-38740.pdf

The extent to which commissioners or analysts can realistically collect this range of data for all client groups will inevitably be limited by the availability of resources:

> There is a real danger ... that data collection continues 'ad nauseam', with enthusiastic researchers chasing after every last publication 'just in case it is interesting'. To avoid this, hypotheses can be helpful, encouraging the data collection to focus on key issues within what could be a very wide field. (Moultrie, 2007)

The challenges involved in the identification and selection of these key issues have been discussed in the section 'The process of developing a strategic needs assessment' and illustrated in Figure 3.2. Some words of caution, however, about the limitations of using data of any sort:

- Most data have varying degrees of uncertainty attached to them and prediction is an uncertain science.
- They can highlight trends and identify particular issues but cannot alone tell you the reasons for them.
- Usefulness of the data and research depends on its robustness.
- Information can vary depending on the time it was collected.

Involving stakeholders

Involving service users, patients and other stakeholders is an important part of putting together an SNA and requires appropriate methodologies. For service users in particular, involvement in the needs analysis is best considered through the two levels of a 'co-production' approach to dialogue – engagement through input and engagement through shared contribution:

Engagement through input

This level involves commissioning and procurement organisations making their existing processes as open to collaboration as possible, and ensuring that active involvement is easy and effective. Commissioners should meet their responsibilities for consultation and partnership collaboratively with enthusiasm and imagination. However, while this level of engagement may well start the process of change and dialogue with stakeholders, it is also challenging. There are excellent examples of the use of video and other social media to aid consultation between citizens and supporting agencies, and these can build up experience and confidence on both sides.

Example activities include:

- Questionnaires to service users, carers and providers asking for comments on needs or services.
- Focus groups exploring views about future requirements.

- Workshops or 'sounding boards' with selected groups of service users to explore the extent to which services meet their needs.
- Advocacy support to facilitate feedback from individuals.
- Reviews of complaints or suggestions schemes.
- Discussions with service users or forums (e.g. youth forums, carer forums, provider forums etc.) to explore their views about service needs
- The use of video and social networking to help citizens produce feedback about services.
- The use of Open Space and Positive Productive Meetings to help support involvement and feedback.

Demand gathering tools like those appearing through systems reviews can also be very interesting.

Engagement through shared contribution

This level involves the recognition that there are many individuals, groups and agencies that have both needs and assets which have the potential to be complementary and mutually beneficial in terms of quality and resource efficiency. This allows the commissioner to transform its typical processes of consultation into communication approaches that support common action and sharing and swapping of assets. Activities might include contributing to the analysis of existing provision, undertaking analysis of future needs, helping to design service specifications or reviewing the impact of services. Certainly this gives commissioners access to a wide group of citizens and groups who increasingly are able to develop common outcomes and are more self-reliant. Importantly they have a better understanding of the interests that they share with the commissioning organisation, its formal responsibilities and the scope of its realistic actions.

Example activities include:

- On-going arrangements for securing regular user, carer and provider input on needs analysis, with feedback to stakeholders on the results of their input.
- Producing a community asset assessment – this can be done collaboratively, with simple web forms with some help to gather the answers verbally for people who do not use the web. The assessment asks agencies, citizens and groups 'what do you need and what can you contribute?' Answers are then collated and the results shared.
- In-depth care pathways and reviews of cases with service users to explore their experience of services, to agree what kind of improvements are needed in the future.

There are significant challenges to both tracks of engagement for commissioners, for example:

- Ensuring that those with learning or communication difficulties are able to make their views understood. The use of a range of media can help, video complaints have proved very empowering, as have big brother diary rooms at events.

- Convincing those who are most vulnerable, and who may rely very heavily on services, that criticism will not have a negative impact on their support.
- Assuring others that their views will have a genuine impact on decisions.
- Ensuring that the sometimes complicated decision-making process in local authorities is understood by those offering their input.
- Ensuring that input is relatively representative of the population of users and carers more widely.
- Recognising the time and energy involved in providing input through some form of token where appropriate.
- Ensuring that those involved in the co-production activity have the right skills and experience to undertake their role effectively – and ensuring that development and training is made available to them.

Database sources

Alongside the above range of methods to create an SNA there are various important online resources. In addition to the Office of National Statistics (ONS) and regional public health observatories some of the other key sources are briefly described below.

Linking the SNA and strategic commissioning

As already indicated an effective JSNA should drive the commissioning process with a perspective on the outcomes commissioners are trying to achieve. To do this the SNA has a range of possibilities in its focus in order to influence commissioning by making the links as strong as possible. The following are suggested as approaches to making these links (IPC, 2010):

- A focus on outcomes
- Reflecting and supporting emerging policy
- Setting commissioning priorities

A focus on outcomes

A strong element that could influence the SNA is the increased focus on what outcomes the public sector can deliver. This approach was emphasised in the original guidance for JSNAs (DH, 2007):

> Historically, most commissioning activity has been expressed through the contractual requirement to provide outputs, such as the number of hours or type of service to be provided. However, measuring the real benefits of services commissioned in this way has proved difficult. In

order to translate priorities into commissioning requirements it will therefore be necessary to consider the outcomes that commissioning bodies want to achieve on behalf of communities.

In terms of the SNA reflecting what an outcomes-based approach to strategic commissioning might look like, it could take some of the high level outcomes for health and local government and explore what data should be captured in order to demonstrate whether those outcomes are being achieved. For example, outcomes identified at a high level for Children's Services have included (HMG, 2003):

- Being healthy: enjoying good physical and mental health and living a healthy lifestyle.
- Staying safe: being protected from harm and neglect.
- Enjoying and achieving: getting the most out of life and developing the skills for adulthood.
- Making a positive contribution: being involved with the community and society and not engaging in anti-social or offending behaviour.
- Economic wellbeing: not being prevented by economic disadvantage from achieving their full potential in life.

Similar outcomes frameworks exist for Personalisation (HMG, 2007), Public Health (DH, 2012) and others. An outcomes-focused SNA would require reviewing the data that can provide information as to whether the themes within the different outcomes frameworks are being achieved or not. It would also want to consider common cause with the outcomes for other public services.

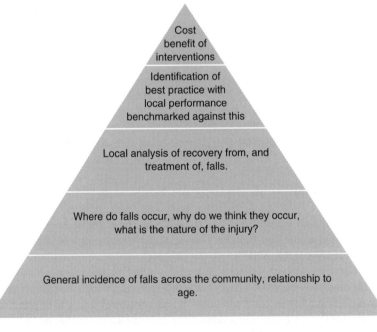

Figure 3.7   A continuum of decision making concerning falls

Stop and Reflect

Take a moment to stop and reflect on your own organisation and its current SNA process.

- If the Government has determined a set of outcomes that it wishes public services to achieve, has the SNA been couched in terms of how well the local community does or does not do in achieving those outcomes?
- Is there clarity in local commissioning strategies about the outcomes that are to be achieved as compared to outputs (the volume and type of service to be delivered) and processes (the activities put in place to ensure services are delivered) and have those outcomes been defined on the basis of the SNA material?
- Is the right balance struck correctly between the need to meet national and local outcomes? Is this explicit? Is it manageable?
- What contribution can SNA authors make to the measurement of outcomes and what may constitute sound and valid approaches?

Reflecting and supporting emerging policy

SNAs do not exist in isolation but have to be completed in the context of the policy changes that affect health and wellbeing – and the public services that promote them. It follows that arrangements for them need to be flexible to take account of these changes. One prominent example is personalisation.

The development of personalisation policies in adult social care may present challenges to the SNA. The original guidance was clear that the SNA was a review of strategic needs as compared to an assessment of individual needs (DH, 2007):

> Needs assessment is an essential tool for commissioners to inform service planning and commissioning strategies. For the purpose of SNA, a clear distinction should be made between individual and population need. SNA examines aggregated assessment of need and should not be used for identifying need at the individual level. Specifically, SNA is a tool to identify groups where needs are not being met and that are experiencing poor outcomes.

For social care the challenge will be considerable. Therefore, although the SNA is not about assessing need at an individual level, in the new climate of personalisation there is a greater requirement for the aggregation of individual data. For example, most authorities would confirm that at present they know little about people who purchase their own health and social care and the relationship of their needs to those who receive state funding. Little is also known about unmet need and yet, as recent reports have revealed (Henwood and Hudson, 2007), often those in social care who fall just below the eligibility threshold have needs which, if unaddressed, may lead to a future demand for public care and support.

What is more, increased personal commissioning may reduce the market influence which public service commissioners have traditionally used as the basis to secure the very services required to deliver the requirements identified in the SNA. Similar considerations will apply as personalisation becomes more widespread across other services and sectors (HMG, 2010).

Stop and Reflect

Take a moment to stop and reflect on your own organisation and its current JSNA process.

- Is there a good understanding of the different and common policy expectations between commissioners and SNA authors?
- Are there agreed methods by which aggregated demand might be collected and analysed including a process for reviewing demand that may not be being met?
- Are there systems locally to capture statutory, independent and voluntary sector supply information and is this used in SNA?
- Does this approach adequately reflect and include the assets of a community?

Setting commissioning priorities

In setting priorities commissioners and SNA authors need to work through a logical sequence starting from a review of the content and development of previous SNAs. Such a review might consider what data was used, why and to what conclusion, the balance between data display and analysis (i.e., was some information included because it had been collected rather than because it led to any conclusion), what areas were included, which were not and why?

If the SNA is to go beyond a broad description of need/demand and begin to address some of the issues which commissioners are most likely to be concerned about, then it needs to have the capacity to understand what those concerns are. Similarly, there is little point in commissioners complaining that the SNA does not meet their needs if they cannot specify what data they would want to have captured and analysed. To change this position commissioners need to be proactively involved in the design of SNAs and SNA authors need to actively invite this to happen.

If there is a changed focus onto commissioning requirements, then the SNA process needs, as argued elsewhere in this chapter, to consider not only the supply side of health and social care but also the relationship between supply and demand. As described previously there is a need to start from a quantitative and qualitative picture of supply to enable comparison between population data and the services that are provided. Part of this picture should also include a review of what

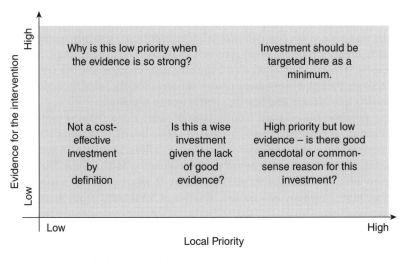

Figure 3.8 Locating priorities (Newbigging and Heginbotham, 2010)

approaches, delivered at what time to particular populations, are likely to have the desired outcomes.

CASE STUDY

Those people suffering poverty, deprivation and health inequality are statistically more likely to suffer domestic violence (DV) although there are no prevalence rates available for domestic violence. In addition there is a tendency for needs assessments to focus on discrete issues that support individual agencies' commissioning agendas with their commissioning decisions being made in isolation. To better address the complex needs of domestic violence sufferers the Nottingham City Local Strategic Partnership looked to reduce this isolation and prevent duplication.

The Local Strategic Partnership (LSP) project aimed to establish linkages from existing data sources across the different agencies to create a picture of those at risk of domestic violence. Additionally, the project looked to gather qualitative information around the 'knowledge on the streets' using a survey with front-line staff and victims of domestic violence.

An initial investigation was carried out into which agencies came into contact with women who were experiencing DV. The main dataset available was police call outs to domestic incidents, which were felt to be quite high. However, it had been identified that there were probably 'cold spots' of reporting. Health staff in particular were identified as uniquely positioned to record prevalence due to the greater likelihood of women attending A&E, being seen by health visitors or attending GP practices after experiencing DV, where the police had not been called out. Recording of DV by different health agencies was investigated and data extracted where

(Continued)

(Continued)

possible. However, given the poor availability of data, a literature review was carried out to identify possible proxy datasets that could be used instead. This identified several factors which indicated increased risk of experiencing DV, including being a single parent, having one or more children, having substance misuse problems, having low income and having mental health problems.

Where possible, the relevant health datasets were extracted and profiled (using a classification methodology) which showed which 'types' of families tended to be overrepresented for the particular indicator, e.g. attendance at A&E with particular injuries, relative to the number of people belonging to that type. These profiles were then used to produce a service framework to identify certain socio-economic groups as 'high', 'medium' or 'low' risk. A series of 'likelihood' maps were then produced which showed for a particular indicator, where over represented types of family lived, therefore indicating where events were likely to occur in future. A combined 'risk of experiencing DV' map was also produced which showed where these over represented family types live, across several indicators. These outputs were shared with the relevant commissioners across the PCT, the CDP (Crime and Drugs partnership) and Children's Services, and also integrated into the DV chapter for the April 2010 update of the Nottingham JSNA.

To address some of the issues around prevalence data gaps identified in the quantitative exercise, focus groups and interviews with health staff and survivors of domestic violence were carried out. This was provided by a local domestic violence qualitative expert. The outcomes were used locally by the DV commissioners in Nottingham to inform planning, training provision, re-configuration of data systems etc.

In conclusion, data sets and linkages were made across LSP members such as the Local Authority, Health, Fire and the Crime and Drugs Partnership. This was enhanced by a 'knowledge on the streets' qualitative methodology and insights were drawn as to how this could be related to other topic areas in terms of capturing staff and service user views.

Source: NHS Information Centre, JSNA Best Practice website at www.ic.nhs.uk

Summary

In this chapter it has been argued that strategic needs analyses have to focus not simply on the needs of individual people or communities or the demand for service, but also on understanding how the market is to provide actual and potential supply into the future. The process of putting together an effective SNA requires the input of all stakeholders including service users and providers. The SNA or JSNA should be at the heart of the commissioning process where commissioners and data analysts are in a constant dialogue about key priorities and questions around commissioning for outcomes.

Further reading and web-based resources

Projecting Older People Population Information (POPPI) Originally developed for the Care Services Efficiency Delivery Programme (CSED), part of the Department of Health, this system provides population data for English local authorities. Available at: www.poppi.org.uk/

Projecting Adult Needs and Service Information (PANSI) Originally developed for the Care Services Efficiency Delivery Programme (CSED), part of the Department of Health, this system provides population data for English local authorities. Available at: www.pansi.org.uk/

Projecting the Care Needs of Wales (Daffodil) Web-based system developed by the IPC for the Welsh Government. Information from research and population projections shows potential need for care over the next 20 years for children, adults and older people. Available at: www.daffodilcymru.org.uk/

Child and Maternal Health Observatory (ChiMat) Specialist Observatory established in 2008 to provide wide-ranging, authoritative data, evidence and practice on child and maternal health. Available at: www.chimat.org.uk/default.aspx

National Adult Social Care Intelligence Service (NASCIS) Provides an array of analytical and information resources. Available at: https://nascis.ic.nhs.uk/Index.aspx

The Network of Public Health Observatories Available at: www.apho.org.uk/

Office of National Statistics Available at: www.ons.gov.uk

References

Cabinet Office (2008) *Think Research*. Cabinet Office Social Exclusion Task Force. London: Policy Research Bureau.

Care Services Efficiency Delivery Programme (2007) *Anticipating Future Needs*. London: Care Services Improvement Partnership.

Department of Health (2007) *Guidance on Joint Strategic Needs Assessment*. London: DoH.

Department of Health (2012) *Improving Outcomes and Supporting Transparency Part 1: A public health outcomes framework for England, 2013–2016*. London: DoH.

Foot, J. and Hopkins, T. (2010) *A Glass Half-full: How an Asset Approach can Improve Community Health and Well-being*. London: IDeA.

Henwood, M. and Hudson, B. (2007) *Cutting the Cake Fairly*, CSCI and Shadow Lands, Young People with a Learning Disability and Eligibility, Voluntary Organisations Disability Group. London: CSCI.

HM Government (2003) *Every Child Matters*. London: HMSO.

HM Government (2007) *Putting People First: A shared vision and commitment to the transformation of Adult Social Care*. London: HMSO.

HM Government (2010) *Equity and Excellence: Liberating the NHS*. London: HMSO.

Humphries, R. and Curry, N. (2011) *Integrating Health and Social Care, Where Next?* London: The Kings Fund.

IPC Institute of Public Care (2010) *Measuring Demand – Making Decisions: A briefing paper exploring the relationship between Commissioning and Joint Strategic Needs Assessment*. North West Joint Improvement Partnership.

IPC (2011) *Co-Production: A way forward for citizen-centred commissioning in Wales*, Briefing Paper for the Welsh Government. Oxford: IPC.

Moultrie, K. (2007) *Developing a Commissioning Strategy in Public Care*. Commissioning e-book. London: CSIP.

Newbigging, K. and Heginbotham, C. (2010) *Commissioning Mental Wellbeing for All: A toolkit for commissioners.* Preston: University of Central Lancashire.

NHS Confederation (2011) *The JSNA: A Vital Tool to Guide Commissioning,* Briefing Issue 221. London: NHS Confederation

NHS Information Centre, *JSNA Best Practice.* Available at: www.ic.nhs.uk/services/in-development/joint-strategic-needs-assessment-jsna/using-this-service/best-practice/nottingham-city)/. Accessed on 6 June 2012

4
Mapping Resources

Maps evoke journeys that are in turn about the possibility of new experience, learning and change. Maps, as the explorer Mark Jenkins (1997) reminds us, can also encourage boldness by making anything seem possible. This chapter is about map making, a set of preparatory activities that complement and develop your assessment as a commissioner of how things are and how things need to be, to give a reasonable idea of the distance involved between these two points and where investment in support including market development may be most critical to the traverse. The approach to travel taken here is not about closing one's eyes and sticking random pins in sheets on the wall as the determinant of direction. Rather this is about deliberate and purposeful enquiry that looks to develop a full understanding of the landscape in front of you. This means that concentrating on the visible and the present will not always be enough. We need to grasp meaning below the surface. We may need to be mindful of histories to explain what it is we see, that this just didn't arrive as it were by accident and to imagine what new elements of future landscapes might look like.

As commissioners we know there is no one right way to map that will fit all needs and circumstances. Rather we have wanted to draw here on experience from a wide range of commissioning programmes and projects to assemble what we think are the basic elements of an effective approach to mapping work. While the detail and mix of these elements will vary from project to project, the evidence does suggest that mapping ideas deployed within large-scale exercises (e.g. 'place-based' approaches) may be readily applicable to smaller scale projects and vice versa. Of course we encourage you to bring your own ideas and expertise to the work.

This chapter introduces some contextual features to the activity of mapping itself, defines that activity and sets out a five-step model to guide its completion. Particular facets of mapping are demonstrated through example including the learning from a case study. Mapping forms a complementary activity to needs assessment and in conjunction with that activity prefaces the planning phases of the commissioning cycle.

Learning outcomes

By the end of this chapter you should be able to:

- Describe the scope and purpose of resource mapping as a key commissioning activity.
- Evaluate your current resource-mapping arrangements against an evidence-informed framework.
- Develop a project plan that is capable of supporting an effective local resource-mapping exercise.
- Draw from a range of mapping techniques to ensure service user perspectives on quality remain central to your mapping work.

Key terms

- *Resources* – goods, services or other assets that may be available to produce individual and social benefits. Resources may be more tangible (buildings, finance) or less tangible (goodwill).
- *Mapping* – a technique to help commissioners identify and locate tangible and intangible resources that either do or could contribute to individual and social benefits within a defined system. Maps as products can take a variety of forms and formats.
- *Co-production* – a reciprocal approach which envisages the public and other sectors and citizens making better use of each others' assets and resources to achieve better outcomes and improved efficiency.
- *Whole systems thinking* – an approach to solution finding that invites us to explore how people, structures and processes interact and influence one another to produce particular outcomes.

Setting the scene – some contextual issues

At first glance, the idea of mapping seems straightforward enough. A closer look, however, at the landscape to be mapped and indeed what constitutes the very idea of 'landscape' suggests that this activity may be more complex than either expected or hoped for. In our experience, setting aside time at the outset of any mapping project to reflect on and address these issues will be time well spent.

In recognition of a broader perspective on what makes a difference to people's lives we use the term 'resource mapping' in this chapter rather than the more traditional idea of 'service mapping'. This of course doesn't dispense with the problems of definition. The question of 'what is a resource?' proves no easier – and indeed may be harder – to answer than 'what is a service?' (see, for example, work by Gatehouse et al. (2008) at the Centre for Child and Family Research on the 'idea' of services for children and families). And what exactly is an 'asset?' These are terms easily used but generally poorly defined in day-to-day activity. As we shall demonstrate, the requirement to be precise about meaning proves to be an essential pre-requisite to decent mapping whether of services, resources or indeed assets.

Services to children and adults have evolved over time and often in an *ad hoc* and opportunistic way into highly complex systems defined as much by local histories as needs and settings. These systems are characterised by a wide range of discrete services and multiple boundaries, which may also function as barriers. One important consequence of this pattern of development is that a holistic picture of needs and contributing influences on outcomes is unlikely to be held by any specific service within the system, i.e. services tend to identify the needs of and outcomes for users through the filter of their own focus of provision. Nevertheless for effective commissioning to occur, understanding this picture, the pattern and nature of this contribution is a prerequisite to reconciling anticipated needs with existing provision, exploring increases in capability within service sectors and identifying critical deficits.

Improving outcomes for children, young people and adults requires services that are well designed, accessible and flexible in the light of local needs and changes to those needs. Improving outcomes overall, however, is not simply contingent on improvements to conventional service provision. Increasingly there is recognition of an equal if not greater role that derives from the building of capacity (or co-production) within communities and families to recognise, accept and assume responsibility for example to improvements in health and wellbeing. It seems likely therefore that claims for the utility and objectivity of mapping activity will be more robust where that activity draws on closer engagement with local communities. Where to draw the boundary around this wider ring of activity and contribution is a necessary albeit not straightforward decision as it inevitably bears on the quality of the final mapping product.

Finally, to have value mapping needs to have purpose. There continues to be evidence that some children, adults and families are offered different levels and standards of care, and that those most in need are not always the most likely to get support. There is evidence that some service users are not accessing services because of local system complexity. We also know that despite some improvement, there continue to be problems of a lack of coherence between the different statutory sectors in coordinated planning and commissioning. This almost certainly compromises the optimum use of finite resources across traditional health, social services and education boundaries. Voluntary sector providers who often play a key role in delivery of services to children and adults are too often left out of the planning and commissioning process. The capability of universal services to respond both earlier and effectively has been historically underdeveloped. The lack of focus on intervening early is associated too often with a tendency for provision to be targeted on high need, higher cost interventions. The lack of early support simply exacerbates the numbers of families who reach crisis point and need more complex interventions.

You've just read at least seven good reasons to undertake some resource mapping activity! There may well be others within your locality. The essential issue here is that the activity has a driving purpose to it. For commissioners, this is often expressed as an idea that by addressing this or that we can do better with the resources available to us than we currently achieve, whether through improved efficiencies, more adaptable services or better outcomes. Effective commissioning relies on building informed hypotheses and testing them with rigour. As the evidence generated by mapping develops it will almost inevitably suggest new directions of enquiry and research – it may even tell you that your original hypothesis left something to be desired. The point is that the need for the journey was recognised and understood and resources mobilised to ensure its completion.

What is resource mapping?

Resource mapping forms part of the 'Analyse' quadrant of the commissioning cycle and is a key activity within it. This activity may have a number of meanings attributed to it and perform a number of functions.

Firstly, it may form part of a *statutory requirement*. So, for example, it is difficult to see how the 1989 Children Act duty on local authorities and partner agencies to identify children in need and make provision for effective services to meet these needs could be satisfied without some essential mapping of the type, location, access criteria, cost and impact of service resources having been made.

Secondly, mapping can be seen as an *intervention* in itself even where the ostensible focus of the activity is the locating of service interventions or 'what works'. That is because mapping activity tends to illustrate to those involved with it the true extent of the actual and potential resources available to a community or to support a particular outcome. In highlighting the true inventory, perhaps for the first time, it will also give rise to ideas about how to demonstrate and disseminate a new picture of our service system. This will be explored in a little more detail in the section on whole systems below.

Thirdly and most commonly, mapping is a collaborative, strategic and iterative *process* for gathering and understanding information on the resources and services available, or potentially available, which an organisation could or might need to mobilise in delivering the outcomes it is seeking to achieve (DfE, 2010). In so doing, mapping activity will identify existing limitations in resources (e.g. gaps, access restrictions/limits) likely to influence strategic improvement.

Resources can include accommodation, workforce (numbers, skills and costs etc.), money (grants, direct payments, charges etc.), assets, and external and internal service providers.

These resources may be under the direct control of the organisation or partnership but, wherever possible, mapping should look to include resources in the wider community, such as those owned by other public bodies and private, voluntary, community or social enterprise bodies. Asset-based approaches take this a step further. Emphasising the kind of principles that underpin notions of co-production, 'asset mapping' is an approach to community development, and refers to a range of approaches that work from the principle that a community can be built only by focusing on the strengths, capacities and capabilities of individual citizens, networks and organisations within a neighbourhood or community. The potential range of these assets is demonstrated in Figure 4.1. Asset mapping emphasises the idea of starting with the positive, for example, what is available from within a community to address the issue or concern rather than starting with a list of what isn't available.

Having this information will provide much greater flexibility when looking at future options for service delivery and efficiencies. It allows you to identify, for example, continuities and gaps in resources and opportunities for working with others to deliver services better, perhaps through grants or sharing of assets. This is very much about a focus on the optimal use of resources strategised to promote better outcomes.

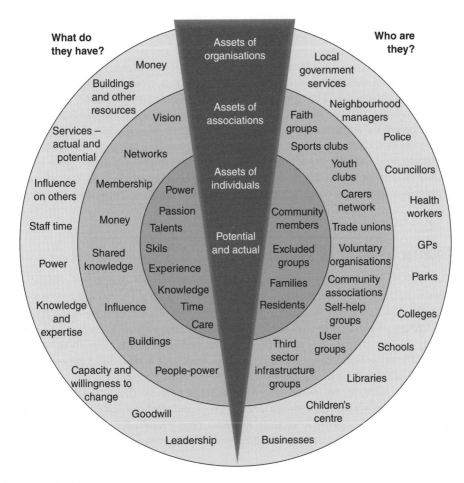

Figure 4.1   Mapping assets

Source: Foot and Hopkins, 2010

Depending on purpose, mapping can focus on known, target or future populations. In any event, mapping activity is rarely complete. Rather maps should be con-
tinually updated as new resources are identified, acquired or developed.

Whole systems approaches

Increasingly, there has been a recognition that the complexity of some needs and the
contributory elements to better outcomes are beyond the gift of a single agency to
meet acting in isolation. They are as Hudson (2006: 6) reminds us 'wicked' problems. Cross-cutting problems like health inequalities and social exclusion are frequently cited examples, but issues like reducing unplanned hospital admissions and
delayed hospital discharges would also be included. In turn these types of challenges
suggest that wider resources (for example community assets) that are beyond the
conventional notion of 'services', will be needed as an integral part of any solution
or response.

This understanding underpins the conceptual approach known as 'whole systems'
and the mapping task that is required to reveal what is often a complex network of
relations and influences. The approach taken here needs to be holistic, collaborative
and inclusive because the parties involved with it will be encouraged to think about
the way the whole service delivery system works, rather than focusing only upon their
own service. Conventional service mapping tends to use an approach that is ultimately
about *separating out individual parts of the system and improving them, often without
reference to one another*. Whole systems thinking by way of contrast focuses on *the
relationship between the various parts of the system* (Hudson, 2006: 8).

Example: Whole systems

The 'Total Place' initiative is one example of an approach to the mapping of public services within a whole area. A central objective here is to obtain better services at less
cost. It seeks to identify and avoid overlap and duplication between organisations,
delivering a step change in both service improvement and efficiency. The process maps
money flowing through the place (from central and local bodies) identifying spend
from different services that contribute to outcomes, and making links between services, to identify where public money can be spent more effectively.

Thirteen pilot authorities considered a wide range of issues that have a direct effect
on people's lives, including children's services, drugs and alcohol misuse, housing, work-
lessness, asset management, services for older people and offender management.
Some of the key learning demonstrated by resource mapping was:

- Confirmation of the complexity of funding streams.
- From the viewpoint of the citizen, public services are often impersonal, fragmented
  and unnecessarily complex.

- Individuals and families with complex needs impose significant costs on areas, but frequently they are currently not tackled through targeted, or preventative activities.

It has also highlighted the true extent of perverse incentives associated with conventional funding and distribution of resources. Late intervention with a young person not in employment, education or training costs four times that of a successful early support package. But unless you have a local concordat, police and probation save that money and health and education spend it. You have to have a place-based budget to be able to handle those kinds of shifts, because local investment streams need to change.

Source: Humphries and Gregory, 2010: 12

Why is resource mapping important?

Resource mapping can be complicated to do and also expensive in terms of thinking and doing time. Below are some value statements that are to do with why mapping activity matters. Think about these in terms of your own commissioning project. The more you can count will probably be an indication that the effort being committed to the task will be worth it. Of course, if at any time the work feels like getting stuck in the sand, you may find it helpful to refer the mapping team (and other stakeholders) back to these statements.

- The history and organisation of care services means that a variety of different agencies will be holding *fragments of a jigsaw rather than a complete picture* (Preston-Shoot and Wigley, 2005: 267). Resource mapping represents a key opportunity for commissioners and key stakeholders to collaborate on developing a shared picture of what there is and what there isn't, what works well and what needs to change.
- Knowledge of existing service provision and its evidence base is essential for effective planning. It is important to be clear about where needs are currently being met, where the gaps and constraints exist before embarking on a process of change. In other words understanding the present allows a better assessment of the likely or expected impact of proposed changes particularly within a whole system perspective.
- Because it is an evidence-informed activity, resource mapping is a key contributory activity to the development of robust design options. The findings from the resource mapping exercise will be important in promoting intelligent decisions on the re-commissioning, decommissioning or redesign of services. This means it forms and informs part of your market shaping and management activities.
- Resource mapping is forward looking and encourages an analysis of the anticipated impact of change within a wide or whole system context. As well as providing a theoretical framework to underpin service provision it will almost always prove to be a source of new ideas. It is certainly difficult to see how more coordinated and cost-effective use of resources can sensibly be achieved without the contribution of mapping.

Stop and Reflect

- How might a whole system asset-based approach to mapping differ from a sector specific service mapping activity?
- What approach seems most helpful to realise the purpose of your project?
- Can you describe the value statements underpinning your mapping project? Who do you need to share and agree these with?

Creating and using a resource map

Commissioners need to have a detailed and comprehensive picture of needs and existing provision within a local authority area. At the same time, mapping should not be so time or resource consuming that it becomes unsustainable. There is, in other words, a need for proportionality, i.e. the quantity of resource applied to any mapping exercise should take account of the size, complexity and priority of the project.

There is no single way to do resource mapping – in fact it will usually involve a combination of approaches. It should also be noted that no community asset map is ever complete – it is a work in progress and will need updating as more and new information becomes available. Mapping will also be about the generation of new perspectives, for example from within services and the community as co-learners and co-creators in the discovery of solutions to the problems that people live with every day.

Providing a census of ongoing activity in a rapidly changing field is a challenge. Results are unlikely to be exhaustive or completely up-to-date. This is due to trade-offs between coverage, the amount of detail that can be obtained, and the likelihood of information becoming dated as new resources come on stream and existing ones end and change. While a 'snapshot', maps provide a valuable and necessary resource for all stakeholders – commissioners, providers, service users and the public at large.

In order to fully realise and sustain the benefits of resource mapping, the best advice is to 'start simple' and look to develop the sophistication and comprehensiveness of mapping over time. It can be helpful to think about and use a stage-based process to your resource mapping project. The following steps are offered as a guide only – you may well want to break them down into smaller elements and the weighting of each will of course reflect local needs and circumstance.

Step one – preparation and planning

Resource mapping can be time consuming and difficult. It therefore needs a clear purpose and rationale. The work is probably best supported by a coordinating team and decent project governance to facilitate the effort. Mapping efforts that do not adequately address these requirements are generally destined to fail.

You also need to begin with agreeing definitions – what are, for example, the need categories and outcomes you want to look at. This will help you to define the potential reach or boundaries to the mapping exercise.

Ideally commissioners need to have good information about all services. Initial attempts at mapping and the allowances you will probably need to make in terms of delivering strategies within realistic timescales and resources, will usually mean some careful targeting of effort. Concentrate most energy on the key priority areas, based on the project boundary and hypotheses identified at the start of the project. However, it won't be helpful to limit the resource analysis to services targeted at the levels of intervention needed to meet the requirements of service users with complex needs. The resources, activities and impact of services at 'lower' levels has to be understood, particularly the extent to which these services are successful in reducing the demand for higher tier interventions.

Stop and Reflect

- What is your hypothesis that resources could be better utilised and coordinated?
- How wide does the review of resources need to be?
- Who is best placed to coordinate the work?

Do ensure that you develop a communications plan to address the information needs of those directly as well as indirectly touched by the focus of mapping activity. You may find that you need to revisit your original scoping for the project, depending on the balance of time investment and anticipated learning benefits that emerge as you progress through the next few steps. This is absolutely fine!

Step two – what information do we need?

This step is about identifying your overall information requirements, together with the approaches, activities and timeline you will use to generate the information.

The information sought should be relevant to the purpose of the mapping, i.e. it should be capable of helping you answer specific questions. These might include:

- What services are currently provided?
- What are the volumes of activity, cost and quality of these services?
- What is the evidence-base informing existing provision?
- Where and how might resources need to be developed or reconfigured to improve outcomes?

You will then need to:

- Identify existing data sources – Is required data already available and how reasonable is its quality? Is there a reliable proxy that can be used?
- Identify new data sources – Consider where retrieval might best be targeted or run a pathway analysis.

Example: Process mapping

Process mapping can be a valuable tool to explore the distribution and location of resources within a care pathway as well as constraints on service delivery and therefore impact on outcomes. It should be an iterative process and one which is capable of reviewing the pathway from a service user perspective.

Needs assessment work or other analyses may indicate particular areas of focus for this activity. Not uncommonly these include:

- High volume service areas.
- High cost service areas.
- High risk service areas.
- Service areas where there is significant variation in practice and variance in outcomes.
- Provision that attracts higher levels of user dissatisfaction.

The mapping activity itself needs to bring all relevant stakeholders together to construct a high level 'as is' map – that is, starting out by understanding how things are before considering how things could be. This will need to start by defining the start and endpoints of the process and then list and sequence all those activities required to achieve existing outcomes in-between these points. It will probably be helpful to use a flow chart with boxes to represent key stages in the process for both the service user and providers. The map at this stage needs to be kept simple and accurate if the analysis that derives from it is to be productive. This high-level process map should:

- Define the sequence of activities.
- Identify the specific responsibility for those activities.
- Define any areas or issues that lie outside the process but will have an impact on it.
- Define the relationships that exist between the different professionals and agencies involved in the process.
- Define potential problem areas or failure points.
- Identify areas where current practice can be improved.

Where service users have not been directly engaged in the mapping activity, process maps should be transcribed and circulated into a process of iterative refinement and review. Once validated, the mapping of future options can start.

The data has to allow a credible, accurate and balanced view of the resource situation although this detail will of course vary greatly depending on the agreed aims of the resource mapping exercise. Ensure relevant data includes outcome measures and unit costs.

You can then begin to refine and complete the dimensions to your mapping framework. This often incorporates a matrix supported by a coding frame to help list and structure information about eligible resources. Figure 4.2 provides an example from a coding frame developed by Aicken et al. (2010) as part of a mapping project concerned with service interventions for childhood obesity. The frame includes five main dimensions together with extensive sub-criteria. Section F of Figure 4.2 is concerned with monitoring and evaluation and covers data collection, follow-up, effectiveness, evidence used to set up the scheme, changes to the scheme and challenges to running of the scheme.

Where you anticipate having to map details of a large or unknown number of services and interventions, particularly within an ambitious timeframe, you will need transparent rules to help with the management of potentially significant amounts of information, for example, through the prioritisation of particular resources.

F.1 *Has monitoring/evaluation data been collected about the intervention?	F.1.1 Yes F.1.2 No F.1.3 Unknown F.1.4 Yes – provided F.1.5 Yes – but not provided F.1.6 In process
F.2 If 'yes', where can this be located? *(please specify)*	F.2.1 Enter details *(free text)*
F.3 *What kind of outcomes are measured in the monitoring/evaluation document? *(select all that apply)*	F.3.1 Changes in BMI F.3.2 Changes in waist measurement F.3.3 Changes in weight F.3.4 Knowledge re: healthy eating F.3.5 Other *(please specify)* F.3.6 Unknown
F.4 In the evaluation/monitoring document, is there any discussion of the main levers and barriers to intervention implementation and effectiveness?	F.4.1 Yes F.4.2 No F.4.3 Unknown
F.5 If 'yes', what are the main levers and barriers identified? *(please specify)*	F.5.1 Main levers *(free text)* F.5.2 Main barriers *(free text)*

Figure 4.2 An example coding frame

Source: Aicken et al., 2010

Stop and Reflect

- What are your essential data requirements?
- What are your rules for including or excluding data?
- How have you reduced bias in your selection of data categories?

Do remember that any research strategy may introduce bias. So for example, if you and your mapping team are predominantly located within the health sector this may mean that interventions provided by teachers or youth workers may be less well known or recognised. It is therefore essential to routinely involve stakeholders from different services and service users themselves in this exercise, as each will bring a different perspective and different local knowledge to it.

Step three – data collection and collation

Having identified your overall information requirements you need to establish the approaches, activities and timeline you will be using to generate the information needed. To gather this information needs patience and resourcefulness, usually involving a combination of activities. You should be prepared to broaden or adapt approaches to collection (desk-top research, telephone surveys, workshops). Different methods will be appropriate to different situations. Individual face-to-face interviews, for example, are likely to be less suited to situations where there are large numbers of target people spread across a wide geographical area. A typical range of activities might include:

- Written questionnaires to existing and potential service providers to gather basic information and provider perspectives.
- Review of spot, block and cost/volume contracts, Service Level Agreements (SLAs) and grants.
- Mapping services by factors such as geographical area, level of need, gender, race or age.
- Finance and budget analysis and projection.
- Interviews and focus groups with service users and carers supplemented by case file reviews exploring impact of provision and feedback from existing user surveys, complaints and compliments system and so on.
- Analysis of some performance indicators or recent service inspections or review.
- Discussions with professionals and advocates working with service users on their views of the service user experience.

Identify all services, locations and resources (for example programme interventions) where needs or outcomes, as defined, are currently met or could be met within the local service system. At this stage you might want to confine the scope of the mapping to two data categories:

- Service descriptor and resource type (Statutory, Voluntary, Private sector)
- Category/categories of need or outcome met by service

Develop a matrix to accommodate this initial set of mapping data. The dimensions to this will be determined by the needs and scope of the mapping project. Figure 4.3 demonstrates a simple but not untypical matrix. This example, developed by Newbigging and colleagues to map women-only day resources, is organised by type and tier of provision on the horizontal axis and by data categories (descriptors) on the vertical axis. Test your scoping and initial results for accuracy with stakeholders. Having established a simple picture of provision across the whole system you can move to the second stage of inputting further categories of information to your matrix. The number, level of sophistication and detail that can be achieved for these categories will depend on:

- The amount of time and resources that can be given to the work.
- The information systems of various local agencies and how comprehensive they are.
- How easy it is to search and retrieve data.

Type of service	1	2	3	4
Description including location/times of operation				
Function				
Function interventions				
No. of places				
Staffing (FTE)				
£ 000				

Figure 4.3 A simple mapping matrix

Source: Newbigging et al., 2006

Stop and Reflect

- What activities will be required to source your data requirements?
- Do you have a sufficient number of descriptors to support your mapping objectives?
- How will you test your data for accuracy?

Step four – analysis

Having collected and collated your basic data set you can begin the process of profiling and analysing the information. The approach to analysing the data will depend on the objectives of the mapping exercise but will routinely involve questions such as:

- How well are the various resources coordinated and integrated?
- Which activities need to be improved or eliminated?
- What's missing?

Aim to look past the statistics to the meaning of the data. Comparing it against reference points such as best practice, statutory requirements, and current and future demand levels will help to reveal their meaning. A typical profile might include:

- The pattern, type, distribution and use of service resources across a continuum of need.
- An understanding of where the key service gaps and constraints are likely to be found.
- A profile of who accesses services – who they are, how and from where and what happens to them on leaving the service.
- A representation of the strength of business activity across a system of provision.
- The distribution of costs across a whole system.
- Where do the outcomes appear to be strongest within the system? Where do they need to be better?
- Are services actually meeting the objectives or delivering the outcomes they say they do, or which users actually want?

Profiling in this way is likely to generate additional questions for you. The answers to these questions will start to suggest where your design priorities should be focused.

Stop and Reflect

- What are the key findings?
- How will these be tested?
- Are there any surprises and what might account for these?

Example: Understanding service quality and impact – the engagement of service users

Virtually all mapping activities will, at some point, need to address the quality of existing provision and use of resources. From both 'co-production' and system design perspectives, it will be important to know that the mapping properly incorporates the status of service users as resource holders rather than passive and potentially grateful service recipients. It is difficult to see how questions of quality can be properly understood or responded to without user views and experience being at the centre of the landscape to be mapped. That is because the questions that have to be addressed at this stage routinely include:

- Are services *accessible* to those who need them – for example are they near enough geographically and easy enough to reach, are there waiting lists for services which mean that potential users are not able to get access when needed, or are the services targeted at the right age group or level of maturity?
- Are services *acceptable* to users – for example does use of the services stigmatise individuals within their local community or peer group, are service users seen positively or negatively by professionals, or do they provide services which users actually want to use to an acceptable standard?
- Are services *effective* – do services actually meet the objectives or deliver the outcomes which they say they do, or which users actually want?

To explore these questions constructively in ways which will be meaningful to stakeholders requires activities which will draw out qualitative themes including:

- Focus group meetings or interviews to explore with them the extent to which professional views of services compare with their own experience.
- Feedback from ongoing user surveys, exit interviews and complaints and compliments systems.
- Analysis of some performance indicators or recent service inspections or review.
- Discussions with professionals and advocates working with service users on their views of the service user experience.

As well as highlighting how particular problems might have emerged, for example in terms of service quality, they will also contribute directly to the practical development of options designed to improve use of resources.

Step five – learning and dissemination

You will now need to engage further with service users, as well as other key stakeholders, to explore and test your findings and their implications for the design of new models or adapted models of service provision across the system. It is the completion of this stage that provides the essential context in which the rationale for change and the shape of that change can best be understood and given legitimacy.

The activity of mapping will itself generate new material. This raises questions about how the mapping information can be best disseminated in a way that facilitates access to the knowledge and resources contained within it. Many public sector organisations utilise Geographical Information Systems to present the links between data and geography to highlight, for example, clusters of activity or non-activity within a given geography. Equally, the information generated by mapping work may well support the production of service and community resources directories. The access needs to mapping information may also vary across stakeholder groups so that consideration will also need to be given to the means (web-based, printed copy and so on) by which material is disseminated as well as content.

Finally this stage should incorporate some useful evaluation of the mapping initiative itself. The focus here is essentially two-fold. Firstly, were the activities identified for the project the right ones, were there specific challenges or difficulties encountered in key tasks and how might these be remedied? Secondly, has the resource mapping achieved its purpose? This may require a longer-term perspective but it is of course of crucial importance that this question is addressed. If we want to say for example that improved outcomes are the ultimate indicator of effective resource mapping, how might this be established? One way may be to compare the results of your next needs assessment with the one you've just completed. In addition, you may want to survey the views and perspectives of those who are affected by the results of the mapping process, for example, service users, professional stakeholders and other community agencies.

Stop and Reflect

- What approach or approaches seem most useful to disseminating the results of your mapping project?
- Are there by-products to the mapping work and how might these best be utilised?
- How will you assess the effectiveness of your mapping work?
- How will you test your findings for accuracy?

Costing services and outcomes: some example approaches

'There is no such thing as a free service' (Local Government Improvement and Development). The following routine hypotheses for commissioners are likely to assume particular resonance during a sustained period of retrenchment.

- It might be possible to use less of a resource and still deliver the same outcomes.
- It might be possible to use different resources that cost less and deliver as good or better outcomes.
- A higher cost service might deliver the results required more quickly making the overall cost cheaper.

To respond with confidence to these or similar hypotheses of course requires tools that support effective and systematic collection and collation of good outcome, service quality and cost data potentially across a whole system of provision. This remains problematic in many areas. Certainly cost measurement of services and interventions across health and social care and public services have conventionally been quite process-driven and service-specific, for example, tending to look only at the direct costs of service provision. Of course many users will be receiving resources from a diverse range of sources. So when calculating costs, it is important to try to think about the indirect costs of service provision to see where true value for money is being achieved and to assess the full public sector impact.

The following short selection of tools is intended to show what the range of potential options looks like. Inevitably but also sensibly, mapping teams will need to consider the utility of these tools in terms of their own project scope and ambition, the extent to which modifications may need to be made to reflect local circumstance and so on.

Acknowledging the difficulties associated with measuring outcomes in a way that allows the costing of their production, the *resource allocation system* (RAS) devised by In Control provides a practical way forward. Using an assessment that provides a scored level of needs and building up local intelligence about local costs, the latest version of this system provides a dynamic framework that can allocate appropriate levels of resources attuned to changing market conditions. RAS is also complemented by POET – the Personal Budgets Outcomes and Evaluation Tool. This tool is the product of a collaboration between In Control and the Centre for Disability Research at Lancaster University.

The *cost calculator for children's services* developed at Loughborough University is a software application that calculates and allows comparison of unit costs for children who are looked after. Analyses of costs with respect to the outcomes variables included in the CCfCS are also available. Development work has started to extend the calculator to children in need and to begin drawing in the costs and contributions made by other agencies within a network of provision. The tool is capable of being adapted for other services.

The Audit Commission's *value-for-money profile tool* is an interactive application that brings together data about costs, performance and activity of local councils. The profiles, utilising a basket of variables, are able to show, amongst other things, how an organisation is spending its resources, and how well services perform; how the costs and performance of an organisation compare to others; outlier reporting. The advice here is to start with high-cost services and analyse cost, quality and outcomes.

Social return on investment (SROI) is an analytic tool for measuring and accounting for a much broader concept of value. It incorporates social, environmental and economic costs and benefits into decision making, providing a fuller picture of how value is created or destroyed.

SROI assigns a monetary figure to social and environmental value that is created. For example, nef (new economics foundation) research on the value created by a training programme for ex-offenders revealed that for every £1 invested, £10.50 of social value was created.

By bringing social and environmental value into decision making, SROI seeks to:

- Reduce inequality, prevent environmental degradation and improve wellbeing.
- Provide a consistent and clear approach to understanding and reporting on the changes caused by an organisation.
- Help organisations improve strategies, systems and accountability.
- Help organisations manage risks, identify opportunities and raise finance required to achieve their mission or strategy.

CASE STUDY

The use of cohorts to understand and analyse types of need and demand for services offers an effective approach to the commissioning of provision over the medium term. The context for the mapping work undertaken within this authority was a relatively high and increasing number of children and young people looked after. The objectives for the work were to provide a trend analysis and to make specific recommendations for resource investment and/or redistribution to meet projected demand.

A cohort approach offers one way to classify and collate a wide range of information in an accessible format. Drawing on the need groups developed by CfCFR for the 'Cost Calculator' and recent work by Hannon et al. (2010) endorsing cost-effectiveness of earlier intervention, a simple four-fold classification was devised:

- Children and families who need early support rather than waiting until they reach crisis point.
- Children who need early permanency as they cannot return home.
- Children who need stability as a permanent solution is not possible or desirable.
- Children and young people who may be able to leave the LAC system through independent living or reunification or other alternatives to care.

The framework proved to be useful in at least three areas of activity.

- Firstly, this high level categorisation was used as a template to enable the mapping and distribution of existing services, to identify areas where provision needed to be strengthened or did not exist at all (see Figure 4.4).
- Secondly, it was used to help organise information about research on effectiveness and best practice in services and to categorise the interventions into one or more of the four groups. This in turn formed the basis to an evaluation of the capacity, capability and purpose of existing provision.
- Finally, the framework could assist the direct and active management of the looked-after population. Resource managers and panels for example could utilise the material organised by cohort so that identified children could access all appropriate interventions according to their circumstance.

To illustrate the utility of the approach, the following are a selection of findings specific to service development that were identified as a result of the resource mapping:

	Children and families who need early support rather than waiting until they reach crisis point	Children who need early permanency (adoption or alternatives to care) as they cannot return home	Children who need stability within looked-after system as a permanent solution is not possible or desirable	Children and young people who may be able to leave the LAC system through independent living or reunification
1. Specialist services (LAC only)				
2. Other specialist services which may include children who are looked after or at risk of becoming looked after				
3. Targeted services including those that may have capability to meet the needs of some looked-after children but have not been established to deal specifically with this group of children				

Figure 4.4   Map of service provision by cohort

- Patterns and projection of demand indicated that the authority needed to strengthen the provision of local fostering resources particularly for younger children.
- No single existing provider had, as its primary purpose, a remit to provide programmes of intensive support to prevent entry of younger children to the looked-after system and/or to enable their exit from it.

(Continued)

(Continued)

- There was evidence of over-capacity within the whole system in terms of provision for needs concerned directly with drug and alcohol misuse. Conversely, provision for children and young people experiencing domestic violence was underdeveloped.
- Eligibility criteria viewed from a whole system perspective was not coherent. This was a factor in the production of service gaps (i.e. services within a pathway not interfacing properly with one another) and constraints or bottlenecks particularly in terms of referral and assessment decisions.
- The service network for all children was complex and poorly understood. This clearly presented to practitioners needing to develop appropriate packages of support involving more than one agency. Information generated by the mapping work should be used to refresh the content of existing service directories.

Summary

This chapter has looked at resource mapping as an essential activity to support good commissioning. It also suggests that for mapping to add real value to your commissioning practice, consideration needs to be given to the contextual and definitional issues associated with any mapping project and that a phased and managed approach to completion is required. By way of a summary, 10 key messages for those about to embark on an exercise or who want to review existing practice are set out here.

- Resource mapping works best if organisations in an area collaborate to carry out the exercise – it will produce a more thorough and reliable picture and distribute costs of the exercise between partners.
- Determine and define the purpose of your mapping activity at the outset, i.e. what is it as a commissioner you are hoping to achieve through this activity? This will help you to be clear about the boundaries to the 'whole system' and inform your priorities where choices about what not to include need to be made.
- Communicate the rationale and objectives for the project to your key stakeholders – what are we doing, why are we doing it, why now and how can you help us?
- Be clear and realistic about the resources you can commit to this activity. You will, at first, almost always underestimate the time, scope and depth of activity involved in mapping single, let alone whole, systems.
- Develop a plan containing an agreed set of activities that are sufficient to cover the scope and ambition for your project.
- Develop a simple framework (for example by tiers of need or provision and cost, location, provider type, outcome indicators) to initially capture, organise and collate your service mapping activity. As mapping expertise develops and the information infrastructure to support it improves, you will be able to extend the scope and sophistication of your mapping activity.
- Start by assembling a relatively small set of measures that are reliable, relevant and useful to provide a profile of whole system activity. Effective mapping is rarely achieved through

the use of quantitative data alone. Make sure you have a reasonable balance of qualitative information to support and complement your analysis.

- Identify the main messages that emerge from your mapping analysis and the explanations that support them. What do these suggest about the design and use of current resources? What appear to be the main implications? Explore, review and if necessary revise these further with stakeholders. Look to obtain a consensual picture – this provides momentum to the process of change.

- Consider what the product of mapping should look like and how best to present the findings. This will vary according to your audience, e.g. formats could include a mix of detailed written reports, newsletters, letters or presentations available as hard copy or web-based materials and so on.

- Document the experience. Make a note of particular areas of difficulty in completing your mapping exercise and take steps to address these where this would help future mapping projects.

Further reading and web-based resources

Care Services Improvement Partnership and Integrated Care Network (2006) *Whole Systems Working: A Guide and Discussion Paper*. This paper is organised into three sections (1) an examination of the factors behind the whole system imperative – why whole systems? (2) an exploration of the question 'what is a whole system?' (3) a review of the issues in managing a whole system together with some illustrations of whole system working in practice. Available at: www.dhcarenetworks.org.uk/_library/Resources/ICN/ICN_Whole_Systems.pdf

HM Treasury (2010) *Total Place: A Whole Area Approach to Public Services*. Provides a summary of the approaches to and learning from 13 pilot sites involved with this initiative. Available at: www.hm-treasury.gov.uk/psr_total_place.htm

Humphries, R. and Gregory, S. (eds) (2010) *Place-based Approaches and the NHS: Lessons from Total Place*. London: The King's Fund. Some useful perspectives on the Total Place initiative from an NHS viewpoint. Available at: www.kingsfund.org.uk/publications/articles/placebased.htm

Newbigging, K., HASCAS and Abel, K. (2006) *Supporting Women Into the Mainstream – Commissioning Women-Only Community Day Services*. Department of Health/University of Manchester. Available at: www.dh.gov.uk/en/Publicationsandstatistics/Publications/PublicationsPolicyAndGuidance/DH_4131070; and

Stevenson, J. (2001) *Mapping Local Rehabilitation and Intermediate Care Services: A Whole Systems Approach to Understanding Service Capacity and Planning Change*. London: Kings Fund. Two good examples of a whole system approach to service redesign and the mapping that was done to support this.

Aicken, C., Roberts, H. and Arai, L. (2010) *Mapping Service Activity: The Example of Childhood Obesity Schemes in England*. London: King's Fund; *BMC Public Health* 10: 31; Available at: www.biomedcentral.com/1471-2458/10/310. Provides details of a specific project concerned with the mapping of resources for children and young people, and helpfully describes the approach taken to the coding and mapping of interventions in larger-scale geographies.

Better Outcomes for Children in Need is a suite of materials written by IPC for the SSIA in Wales and designed to improve local arrangements for the commissioning of children's services. The Resource Book contains tools to support resource mapping and understanding service quality and impact and can be accessed at www.ssiacymru.org.uk/media/pdf/g/b/ BOCIN_-_Complete_document.pdf

Foot, J. and Hopkins, T. (2010) *A Glass Half-full: How an Asset Approach can Improve Community Health and Wellbeing*. London: IDeA. UK-based example of the use of asset-based approaches to resource mapping.

A useful overview of tools to support financial aspects of mapping can be found on the 'cost and value for money' pages of the Local Government Improvement and Development website. Available at: www.idea.gov.uk/idk/core/page.do?pageId=7989471. This also includes links to:

- *Resource allocation system* (RAS) devised by In Control. Available at: www.in-control.org.uk/support/support-for-organisations/resource-allocation-systems-(ras).aspx
- *The cost calculator for children's services.* www.ccfcs.org.uk
- *Extension of the Cost Calculator to Include Cost Calculations for all Children in Need* (Research brief DFE-RB056, 2010) prepared by Holmes et al. at the Centre for Child and Family Research, Loughborough University, reports on the results of mapping activity designed to support the costing of services to children in need. Available at: https://www.education.gov.uk/publications/RSG/Childrenand families/Page8/DFE-RB056
- The Audit Commission *value-for-money profile tool*. Available at: http://vfm.audit-commission.gov.uk/
- *Social return on investment* (SROI). Available at: http://neweconomics.org/publications/guide-social-return-investment

Graves, B.A. (2008) 'Integrative literature review: A review of literature related to geographical information systems, healthcare access, and health outcomes', *Perspectives in Health Information Management*, 5(11):1–12; and

Foley, R. (2002) 'Assessing the applicability of GIS in a health and social care setting: Planning services for informal carers in East Sussex, England', *Social Science & Medicine*, 55(1): 79–96. GIS provides a powerful way of presenting a link between data and geography. These two papers are drawn from the adult health care sector but do show the scope of this technology to support mapping activity more generally.

References

Aicken, C., Roberts, H. and Arai, L. (2010) 'Mapping service activity: The example of childhood obesity schemes in England', *BMC Public Health*, 10: 310. Available at: www.biomedcentral.com/1471-2458/10/310

Department for Education (2010) *How to Map Resources*. Available at: www.education.gov.uk/childrenandyoungpeople/strategy/a0065946/procurementskills

Foot, J. and Hopkins, T. (2010) *A Glass Half-full: How an Asset Approach can Improve Community Health and Well-being*. London: IDeA.

Gatehouse, M., Ward, H. and Holmes, L. (2008) *Developing Definitions of Local Authority Services and Guidance for Future Development of the Children in Need Census*. Research Report DCSF – RW033. Loughborough University.

Hannon, C., Wood, C. and Bazalgette, L. (2010) *In Loco Parentis*. London: DEMOS.

Hudson, B. (2006) *Whole Systems Working: A Guide and Discussion Paper*. Care Services Improvement Partnership (CSIP) and Integrated Care Network (ICN).

Humphries, R. and Gregory, S. (eds) (2010) *Place-based Approaches and the NHS. Lessons from Total Place*. London: The King's Fund.

Huxley, J. (1957) 'Transhumanism' in *New Bottles for New Wine*. London: Chatto & Windus.

Jenkins, M. (1997) *To Timbuktu*. New York: William Morrow & Co.

Local Government Improvement and Development 'How do you know services are cost effective and provide value for money?' Available at: www.idea.gov.uk/idk/core/page.do?pageId=7989471. Accessed 10 May 2012.

Newbigging, K., HASCAS and Abel, K. (2006) *Supporting Women into the Mainstream*. Department of Health/University of Manchester.

Preston-Shoot, M. and Wigley, V. (2005) 'Mapping the needs of children in need', *British Journal of Social Work*, 35(2): 255–275.

Section 2

Plan

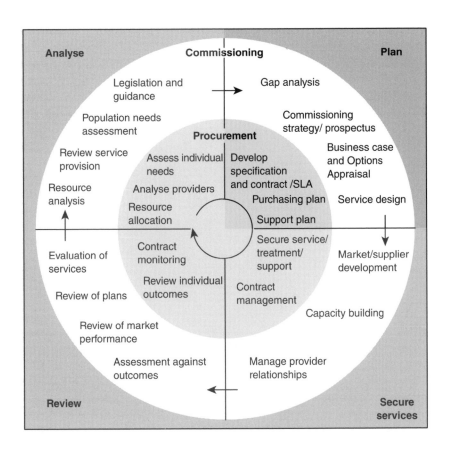

5

Strategic Analysis Tools for Commissioning

The next two chapters both look at the 'why' and 'how' of developing a commissioning strategy for public care services and at some of the tools which can be used to support a sysytematic analysis to underpin the commitments made in a strategy.

A commissioning strategy is a strategic statement about how an organisation intends to specify, secure and monitor services to deliver particular outcomes for citizens. In developing a strategy, commissioners take account of national and local drivers in articulating the outcomes to be achieved for particular populations and sub-populations.

The strategy needs to describe the service model(s) that are to be commissioned and will indicate how their effectiveness will be monitored and measured. It will include high-level cost information.

Learning outcomes

By the end of this chapter you should be able to:

- Understand the purpose of a commissioning strategy.
- Understand the processes involved in strategy development.
- Conduct a cost benefit and risk analysis, social return on investment and multi-criteria analyses as part of the analysis involved in developing a strategy.

Key terms

- *Commissioning strategy* – a set of high level, long term goals describing how you are going to effect change in the overall configuration of services across a market to meet the needs of the whole population. High level information about cost will be included.
- *Outcome* – the desired positive result or impact of the commissioned service for the service user (individual level outcome) or the population as a whole (strategic level outcome).
- *Output* – the amount of services produced in a given time.
- *Processes* – the ways of working put into place to achieve the outputs.
- *Inputs* – the resources needed to deliver the outputs.
- *Business case* – an approach to reviewing services and identifying options for change in line with priorities identified within the strategic commissioning strategy.
- *Option appraisal* – a document which outlines objectives; the possible options for delivering the objectives and reviews the relative benefits and costs of the options.
- *Market position statement* – a market-facing document bringing together data from the joint strategic needs assessment, commissioning strategies, and market or customer surveys, into a single document to inform and be of benefit to the provider sector.

What is a commissioning strategy?

A commissioning strategy is one way of describing priorities for an area or population. It is a statement of intent to guide those designing, providing and using services. It is based on a rigorous analysis of information and data gathered during the analysis stage of the commissioning cycle.

Stop and Reflect

- What are the current strategic priorities in your local area or organisation?
- How do these relate to the specific population outcomes with which you work?

What is the value of a commissioning strategy?

A commissioning strategy has a number of key functions:

- To support the communication of the strategic vision and priorities to stakeholders.
- Developing joint or aligned commissioning processes can help agencies work more effectively together.

- To address needs of users and client populations in an integrated way.
- Having clear long term goals helps to navigate through any immediate funding crises.
- To give a clear link between service development, business cases and investment plans.
- To enable on-going review of all service provision.
- To provide an evidence base for decision making.
- To ensure all providers (in-house, direct and external) are treated on the same basis.

Stop and Reflect

- Do you agree with this list of functions?
- Would you add anything to this list?

The process of developing a commissioning strategy

Figure 5.1 provides a way of thinking about the processes involved in developing a commissioning strategy. It contains five stages and takes the commissioner from gathering and analysing data to writing a strategy (CSIP, 2007).

In Stage 1 baseline data is collected. The data looks at both supply and demand. At the same time policy guidance and legislation are identified and related to the commissioning activity.

In Stage 2 the data is analysed and any gaps in information identified. Further information may be gathered through a review of research and best practice. Additionally, small, local research projects may be conducted to help provide further information.

Stage 3 uses the information gathered in the previous two stages to map possible service design options against demand.

Stage 4 provides an analysis of the costs and implications of the proposed service models. The proposals are subject to consultation, particularly with service users.

In the fifth and final stage the data and analysis are pulled together and the commissioning strategy needs to be produced and agreed by all of the key stakeholders and budget holders involved.

What should be in a commissioning strategy?

Commissioning strategies can vary in their level of detail, depending on their purpose and relationship to other strategic documents. In IPC's experience, however, there are some standard basic elements of a strategy which are needed to ensure that the strategy is usable, relevant and useful to those who need to implement it.

A commissioning strategy will need to contain the following:

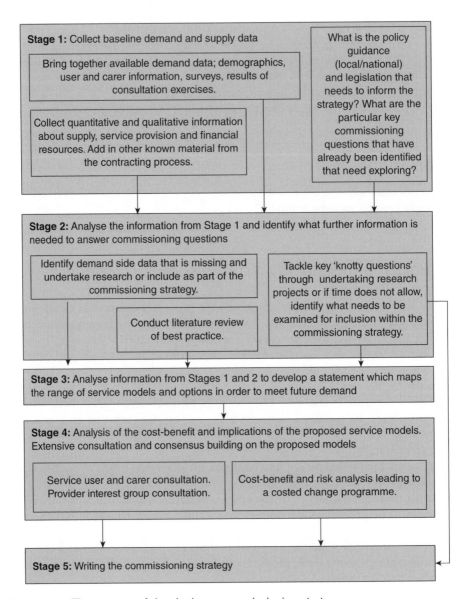

Figure 5.1   The process of developing a commissioning strategy

1. **Executive Summary**

The Executive Summary gives an overview of the strategy, the agreed approach, the timescales and the investment/disinvestment to be made over that period. It can be produced as a separate, short document, or as a summary at the front of the strategy.

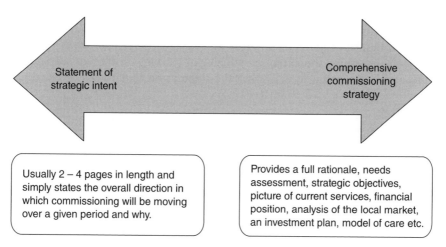

Figure 5.2 Commissioning strategy spectrum, IPC

Source: Institute of Public Care

2. Introduction

The introduction describes the purpose of the strategy and the values/vision informing it. It provides a brief picture of the service area under consideration and identifies the priorities and the outcomes that the strategy is trying to achieve. There may also be a brief description of how the strategy was developed.

3. National and Local Guidance and Research

This section contains an overview of the major policy issues both locally and nationally. It will emphasise the key drivers for change, highlighting any essential actions required by legislation, national guidance or local commitments.

4. Demand Analysis

This section provides an analysis of the needs of the relevant population and how these are likely to change in future. It provides a robust but focused analysis to help illustrate the purpose and objectives of the strategy.

5. Supply Analysis

This is an analysis of current and potential services and resources and the extent to which they are likely to meet future needs.

6. Gap Analysis

This shows the strengths and limitations of current services, the changes needed, and some detail about the types of services which will be commissioned. It also highlights the types of service which will not be commissioned in future.

7. **Monitoring and Review**

The section describes plans to monitor and review the impact of the strategy. It will seek to determine the extent to which the strategy is shaping service design/delivery and is successful in delivering the population outcomes identified.

8. **Appendices**

These may include:

- A contracting or procurement plan.
- A market position statement.
- The full results from the demand/strategic needs and the supply side assessment.
- Results of consultation exercises.
- All key performance indicators and other important indicators appropriate to the population.
- A glossary of terms used in the strategy.
- Key research and guidance documents.

Stop and Reflect

- How might you use this planning template in your day to day work as a commissioner?

Specific tools and methodologies to support the strategic analysis

Gap analysis

A gap analysis establishes the gaps between identified needs (obtained from the needs analysis) and existing provision (obtained from the market analysis). It helps to answer two questions: where are we now and where do we want to be?

The following activities are used to carry out a gap analysis:

- A review of the data collected during the needs analysis about the nature, extent and location of service need.
- A review of the data collected during the market analysis about the extent to which services currently meet those needs and are likely to meet them in the future.
- A review of quality and consultation data about what sorts of services are most effective and efficient, and whether these types of services are currently being delivered.

The data helps to answer a set of questions, such as:

- Are there any gaps in particular types of services?
- Is there an absence of service within a particular community?

- Are some services weak or of poor quality?
- Are some services in inappropriate locations or inaccessible?
- Is there an over-provision of particular services?
- Is there an over-provision of services within particular communities?
- Is the funding for particular services sustainable?

Gap analysis template

Commissioners can use the following template to help them draw together the types of data identified in the previous section. The template can be gradually populated from left to right, with the rationale for the proposed service developments completed with the evidence gathered during the analysis activities, and the commissioning implications developed from the consultation activities. In this way the thinking behind commissioning objectives can be shared with stakeholders as it is developed.

In the following worked example a local authority has been investigating the use of day care services, and whether there are more effective and cost-effective ways of providing community support for service users and their carers.

Strategic Objective	The Gap – Service Developments	Rationale	Commissioning Implications
Describes the overall outcomes intended for the population. 7–8 maximum. Derived from the organisation purpose, legislation, national guidance. 5–10 year timescales.	Specific service developments needed to meet strategic objectives. Based on the evidence collected in the needs analysis. Which patients/service users the service developments are for. Where the services are needed. 2–3 year timescales.	Why the service developments are needed, based on guidance, research, needs, service and market analysis. Why existing arrangements will not meet user/carers' needs in the future.	Disinvestment/ decommissioning, remodelling or renegotiation required. Procuring and contracting with providers. Redistribution of resources required. Interim/transition costs.

Figure 5.3 Gap analysis template

Scenario

In this imaginary scenario, the analysis revealed a very high proportion of service users who did not value existing day services. There were a high number of places that were not taken up by service users, the unit cost of provision appeared particularly high in the north of the area, and a large proportion of carers interviewed said they wanted social care support to be made available in their own home. In this case the template might start to look like Figure 5.4.

Strategic Objective	The Gap - Service Developments	Rationale	Commissioning Implications
To re-configure day care support for older people with no medical support needs, to better meet their social care needs, and support carers more effectively.	Introduce a scheme to provide home-based support for older people who are supported by single carers in the north of the area.

Revise the role and remit of the existing day centre to support only those with combined health and social care needs. | Feedback from existing service users and carers and staff that day centres are not meeting the needs of a significant proportion of existing users.

Cost and unit costs data show service inefficiencies.

Examples from other authorities and research showing that alternative, home-based provision can be more effective in meeting the needs of people supported at home by a single carer.

Existing providers and potential new providers have expressed interest in preparing proposals for alternative services. | Change the eligibility criteria for day centres and reduce the number of available day centre places in the north of the area.

Reduce the funding for the existing day centres.

Specify requirements and invite tenders from potential providers of home based support.

Evaluate the impact of the scheme, with a view to introducing further changes elsewhere in the following two years. |

Figure 5.4   Example gap analysis template

Following consultation, the gap analysis might be followed by an exercise with a range of stakeholders to design the service model for home-based social care support, and to test out how the service might be delivered in a range of scenarios.

Stop and Reflect

- How helpful would this sort of template be to you in conducting a gap analysis?

There are many different approaches to preparing and presenting a systematic analysis of the range of complex data collected and completing an options appraisal in the course of developing a commissioning strategy. In the sections below three of the most popular approaches are considered.

Option appraisal should help to develop a value for money solution to meet the objectives of a strategy. An effective option appraisal will usually include an assessment of:

- Strategic option casts.
- Benefits and risks.

- Whether the strategic option benefits are worth the cost and the risk.
- The best strategic option that will deliver the desired outcomes, at the right time and at an acceptable cost and level of risk.
- Whether there is adequate baseline information to allow the strategy to be evaluated.

The *Green Book* (HM Treasury, 2003) recommends that option appraisal should take place wherever practical, but that it should be proportionate to the proposals in question.

There are three particular techniques which can be used by commissioners and managers to support and strengthen option appraisals, decision making and evaluation: cost benefit analysis (CBA); social return on investment (SROI); and multi-criteria analysis (MCA).

Cost benefit analysis

Cost benefit analysis (CBA) is a useful approach for anyone required to do a basic option appraisal, allocate resources or evaluate a policy, project or programme. It is a key tool for commissioners in relation to drawing up strategic business cases and deciding how to redesign systems to:

- Reduce inefficiencies.
- Improve quality.
- Decommission services.

Cost benefit analysis quantifies and expresses the costs and benefits of a service or programme in the context of today's money, including items which do not normally have a monetary value. Decisions are based on whether there is a net benefit or cost to the service, that is, total benefits less total costs.

CBA can be essential in setting out the costs and benefits associated with different options, and in making a rigorous choice between them. However, it is rarely sufficient on its own, because other, often more nebulous, factors will also need to be taken into account. The option identified as 'best' from a CBA does not always need to be chosen – but any departure from the 'best' option needs to be very carefully justified.

Basic steps

The key stages of CBA are:

- Establish rationale for action (understanding the need for the intervention and what would happen if it wasn't put in place).
- Set the objectives for the intervention.
- Identify options, drawing on best practice, demographics, market context and consultation, including a 'do minimum' option.

- Estimate costs including fixed, variable and external costs.
- Estimate the value of benefits (and external benefits).
- Value costs and benefits where there is no market value.
- Adjust for distributional impacts, for example, inequality of impact on vulnerable groups.
- Adjust for relative price changes, for example, technology, fuel prices.
- Adjust for bias, risk and uncertainty.
- Compare costs and benefits of different options.
- Present the results.

Resources required

The resources required for a CBA may vary according to scale and complexity of the service or intervention and the level of detail needed. A degree of financial expertise is needed to carry out some of the financial calculations, for example, net present value of investment and other aspects of the valuation process.

Examples

Many examples of CBA relate to large-scale capital projects; however, there are a growing number from the world of public care, for example:

- Research into the financial benefits of investment in specialist housing for vulnerable and older people by Frontier Economics for the Homes and Communities Agency in 2010 concluded that the total benefit of specialist housing was about £1.6bn. The researchers identified a £990m incremental cost of providing that housing, over-and-above the alternative. This suggested a net benefit of about £640m. The largest single benefit was estimated for the older people client group. There were also significant positive benefits for people with mental health problems and people with learning difficulties.

Strengths

As a means of supporting an option appraisal, CBA has a number of strengths. A CBA:

- Forces disciplined consideration of choices, including the status quo option.
- Recognises that each choice has a cost (however unpleasant that admission might be).
- Makes hidden costs and benefits explicit.
- Is objective in the sense that it follows an established and open methodology.
- Forces more detailed consideration of what we mean by the adjectives placed in front of the word 'value' (e.g. societal, cultural, etc.).
- Overcomes 'programme optimism' – the tendency of project appraisers to be over-optimistic.

Weaknesses

The potential weaknesses or pitfalls of CBA are:

- The possibility of missing out some key options, or some key costs and benefits. If this occurs, the results of the analysis can be significantly skewed away from the actual 'best' option. This underlines the need to take time to make an exhaustive list of the options, and all the different costs and benefits that could arise – even if some are later excluded.
- An over-reliance on the quantitative data. In practice, CBA rarely gives proper recognition to qualitative and non-market factors, such as equity, quality of life and the like.
- Valuation techniques are imperfect and loaded with assumptions. The parameters and any underlying assumptions about costs, benefits, risks and discount rates need to be clearly defined and transparent.
- Information on costs, benefits and risks is rarely known with certainty, especially when one looks to the future. This makes it essential that sensitivity analysis is carried out, testing the robustness of the CBA result to changes in some of the key numbers.
- Wherever possible, CBA should be carried out collaboratively across agencies in order to assess fully the benefits and costs to different stakeholders with clear links with commissioning strategies. In the case of health and social care, this can be difficult.

Conducting a social return on investment (SROI) analysis

Social return on investment (SROI) has its roots in cost benefit analysis and social accounting. The approach can be used by private, public sector and VCS organisations and is appropriate for both large and small organisations to improve performance, inform expenditure and highlight the value they add. Commissioners and funders may use the approach to secure value for money by using it during strategic planning, to assess tenders, and for contract management.

SROI is a framework for measuring and accounting for a much broader concept of value than just money. It incorporates social, environmental and economic costs and benefits, and helps organisations to understand better the economic value that they create by assigning a monetary value to all these factors. For example, NEF research on the value created by a training programme for ex-offenders revealed that for every £1 invested, £10.50 of social value was created.

SROI is underpinned by seven principles that are core to the approach:

- Involve stakeholders
- Understand what changes
- Value the things that matter

- Only include what is material
- Do not over claim
- Be transparent
- Verify the result

There are two types of SROI:

- *Evaluative SROI*: undertaken retrospectively and based on actual outcomes that have taken place over a given period. This approach is best used when a project has been set up and good data on outcomes are available.
- *Forecasted SROI*: predicts how much social value will be created if planned activities meet their intended objectives. Forecasted SROIs can be used at the planning stages of a project to assess its likely impact, or for projects where there is a lack of outcomes data.

A forecasted SROI can be followed by an evaluative SROI once the project has been implemented to assess the accuracy of the predictions.

Basic steps

There are six stages to SROI:

- Establish scope and identify stakeholders and how to involve them.
- Map outcomes, linking the relationship between inputs, outputs and outcomes.
- Evidence outcomes and give them a value – find data to show what outcomes have been achieved and decide what value they have.
- Establish impact and clarify which aspects are directly related to the project/programme.
- Calculate the SROI – consider both negative and positive benefits to arrive at a total value.
- Reporting, using and embedding the results.

Resources required

The length of time and resources it takes to carry out an SROI varies significantly depending on the scope of the analysis and the extent to which outcomes data are already available. SROIs can be done in-house or the SROI Network has details of accredited SROI practitioners.

Questions to consider when establishing the resource requirement include:

- Is the analysis for external publication or to inform management decisions?
- What is the size of the project or organisation?
- What is the availability of data and research on outcome?
- Is a forecasted or evaluative SROI required?
- What skills do staff have to undertake an SROI?

Strengths

SROI has many uses and some of the strengths of the approach can be described as follows:

- Can be used to develop public policy when social value is important.
- Facilitates decision making and strategic discussions and helps to identify the social value of activities.
- Demonstrates the importance of partnership working and that the impact of change may be much wider than an individual project.
- Aids strategic planning by allowing a wider view to be taken of the potential impact of projects or activities.
- Encourages engagement and commitment by a wider range of stakeholders.
- Highlights both potential negative and positive outcomes so that corrective action can be taken.
- Can improve the case for funding and investment and make tenders more convincing by creating a wider interpretation of 'return on investment' and provides a better understanding of value for money.

Weaknesses

The limitations of using SROI include:

- It is very difficult to translate some benefits and outcomes in commissioning into a monetary value, for example, increased self esteem.
- If an organisation seeks to monetise its impact, without having considered its mission and stakeholders, there is a risk of choosing inappropriate indicators. As a result, the SROI calculations can be of limited use and miss the real difference that a service makes to people's lives.
- The approach can be very resource intensive when used for the first time, particularly if outcomes data are not available. It is most easily used when an organisation is already measuring the direct and longer term results of its work with people, groups or the environment.
- The focus of the methodology is on outcomes and therefore may ignore processes which affect the quality of the user experience.
- A diverse skill set is required from staff using the methodology.

Multi-criteria analysis

Multi-criteria analysis (MCA) provides a framework to enable decision makers to overcome difficulties in handling large amounts of complex information in a consistent way. It provides a structured process for determining both the criteria by which a range of options will be assessed, and the relative importance of each of the criteria. This enables a single preferred option to be identified. The judgement of the decision-making team in establishing explicit objectives and criteria, scoring and weighting is a critical feature.

MCA and multi-criteria decision analysis (MCDA) provide a way of looking at complex problems that have a mixture of monetary and non-monetary objectives, where defining monetary values for costs and benefits is impractical or not very robust, and where there are non-monetary items that may be of major importance.

They can be used to:

- Identify the single most preferred option.
- Prioritise or rank options.
- Clarify the differences between options.
- Indicate the best allocation of resources to achieve objectives.
- Improve communication between stakeholders.

Multi-criteria analysis establishes preferences between options by reference to an explicit set of objectives agreed by the decision-making group, and for which the group has agreed measurable criteria to assess the extent to which objectives have been achieved. Typically there may be 6 to 20 criteria – which may be grouped. Criteria need to capture the key aspects of the objectives, be applicable in practice, relevant and discrete.

The key tool is the development of a 'performance matrix' where each row describes an option, and each column the performance of the options against each criterion. This can be the final product of the analysis, leaving the decision makers to assess the extent to which their objectives are met by the entries in the matrix.

When the performance matrix is completed, any options which perform weakly can be ruled out. There may be trade-offs between different criteria, so that good performance on one criterion compensates for weaker performance in another.

Basic steps

There are five key steps in MCA:

- Establish the decision context: what are the aims of the analysis, who are the decision makers, and other stakeholders?
- Identify the options.
- Identify the objectives and criteria to be used to compare options, e.g. coverage, cost, availability of alternative service.
- Describe the expected performance of each option against the criteria.
- Examine the results, make choices.

Multi-criteria decision analysis (MCDA) involves two further stages:

- Scoring expected consequences of each option on a scale, often from 0 to 100.
- Weighting the relative value of each criterion (and how much the difference matters).

One overall value is obtained by multiplying the value score on each criterion by the weight of that criterion and then adding those weighted scores together. A sensitivity analysis can look at the results of changes to scores or weights.

Resources required

The resources required for MCA will depend on the scope and complexity of the analysis. Skills in facilitation are needed to enable the decision-making team to identify and agree objectives, criteria and how objectives will be measured at the start of the MCA, and to decide how to apply scores and weight the performance matrix later in the process.

Strengths

MCA has a number of strengths:

- It can incorporate a wider range of criteria (e.g. social, ethical, environmental) than a typical financial analysis, and unlike a cost-benefit analysis, does not require monetisation of all costs and benefits.
- It brings a systematic approach to appraising and comparing options with a wide range of quantifiable and non-quantifiable impacts.
- Open and explicit: the choice of objectives and criteria are open to analysis and change if they are felt to be inappropriate.
- Flexible in terms of: choice of options, criteria, weighting, and who is involved.
- Develops shared understanding among decision-making group of objectives, options, criteria, weighting and scoring.
- Provides an audit trail, especially in situations where decision making is required to follow rules and to be justified in explicit terms.

Weaknesses

The weaknesses of MCA include:

- Lacks the methodological rigour of CBA and linkage to commissioning strategies.
- Based on decision makers' own choices of objectives, criteria, weights and assessment of achieving objectives – makes them explicit, but embeds subjectivity.
- Cannot show that an action adds more to welfare than it detracts.

- Weighting and scoring introduce additional stages to the process and make it less transparent.
- Weighting may be hard to derive.

Stop and Reflect

Read the following scenario:

A large unitary authority, Betterton, has decided to review its range of provision for adults with learning disabilities, as a result of a lower financial settlement due to an economic downturn and an increasing number of adults with learning disabilities requiring social care support. Betterton wants to set a 10 year strategy for learning disability services which is both efficient and high quality. The authority needs to understand the levels of future demand and the different range of service models it could consider.

- Which approach to options appraisal would you use and why?

This case study describes how a Substance Misuse Partnership (SMP) in a large urban area developed a commissioning strategy.

The strategy was aimed at a specific part of the city where, due to the daily influx of workers, the resident and day-time population differed both in number and need.

Initially a steering group was established and a range of stakeholders was seconded onto it. One of the first tasks of the group was to take an honest and open look at data describing need in the area. This analysis demonstrated that the substance misuse of the daily influx of workers was significant and different in scale from that of the resident population. This prompted the steering group to engage with other stakeholders from the business community.

At the same time the relevant national drivers changed; for example, the Health and Social Care Bill (2011) and the National Drugs Strategy (2012). The National Drugs Strategy re-focused funding and provision from harm reduction to recovery.

The strategy sets out a 3–5 year outcomes-based plan for the commissioning and delivery of services to problematic drug and alcohol users for both the area's small residential population, and its much larger working and visiting population. It is informed by the drivers of cost reduction, and choice and personalisation in public services. It also emphasises the need for collaborative working across agencies and political boundaries.

The strategy first assesses the legislative and policy context by which the new strategy must be driven, including the financial implications of the annual Comprehensive Spending Review and also service reconfigurations such as the momentum towards localism and greater community empowerment.

It then performs separate needs assessments for drug and alcohol services, in light of the area's very particular demographic context, and reviews existing services. These are found to be broadly responsive and well integrated, but areas for development to meet the personalisation agenda are identified, including the need for a system of individual budgets and a wider variety of treatment options, in which context the strategy also emphasises the need for a market development plan.

Current financial and staffing resources are assessed, and a risk assessment performed that highlights in particular the potentially destabilising effects of internal reorganisation and uncertainty over ongoing funding. The strategy also sets out plans for monitoring and review, using a balanced scorecard method to measure the impact of proposed service changes.

Finally, key priorities for the strategy are summarised.

Stop and Reflect

- How could you make use of this approach to strategy development to help deliver strategic priorities in your own context?

Summary

A commissioning strategy is a statement indicating how an organisation intends to specify, secure and monitor services to deliver particular outcomes for citizens. It is developed by a process of gathering and analysing supply and demand data, articulating a statement of intent and evaluating the options that will deliver the desired outcomes in the most efficient and effective way. You have had the opportunity to consider specific tools and methodologies and their possible use in your own context.

Further reading and web-based resources

http://ipc.brookes.ac.uk

Prime Minister's Strategy Unit (2004) *Strategy Survival Guide*. Available at: http://interactive. cabinetoffice.gov.uk/strategy/survivalguide/skills/ao_cost.htm

Fujiwara, D. (2010) *The Department for Work and Pensions Social Cost-Benefit Analysis Framework: Methodologies for Estimating and Incorporating the Wider Social and Economic Impacts of Work in Cost-Benefit Analysis of Employment Programmes*, DWP Working Paper No. 86. London: DWP. Available at: http://research.dwp.gov.uk/asd/asd5/ report_abstracts/wp_abstracts/wpa_086.asp

A Guide to Social Return on Investment (2012) Available at: www.neweconomics.org/sites/ neweconomics.org/files/A_guide_to_Social_Return_on_Investment_1.pdf

Measuring What Matters. London: Cabinet Office/Centre for Public Scrutiny. www.cfps.org. uk/what-we-do/publications/cfps-general/?id=148

Scholten, P., Nicholls, J., Olsen, S. and Galimidi, B. (2006) *SROI A Guide to Social Return on Investment*. Amsterdam: Lenthe Publishers.

Nicholls, J., Mackenzie, S. and Somers, A. (2007) *Measuring Real Value: A DIY Guide to Social Return on Investment*. London: New Economics Foundation.

nef (the new economics foundation). Available at: www.neweconomics.org

Social Return on Investment Network. Available at: www.thesroinetwork.org/

SROI project (Scotland). Available at: www.sroiproject.org.uk/

European SROI network. Available at: www.sroi-europe.org/

Proving and Improving. Available at: www.proveandimprove.org/new/tools/sroi.php

SROI primer. Available at: http://sroi.london.edu/

Social Return on Investment position paper (New Philanthropy Capital). Available at: www.philanthropycapital.org/publications/improving_the_sector/charity_analysis/sroi_position_paper.aspx

Local Government Improvement and Development. Available at: www.idea.gov.uk/idk/core/page.do?pageId=23233317

Department for Communities and Local Government (2009) *Multi-criteria Analysis: A Manual*. London: DCLG.

Prime Minister's Strategy Unit (2004) *Strategy Survival Guide*. Available at: http://interactive.cabinetoffice.gov.uk/strategy/survivalguide/skills/ao_multi.htm

References

CSIP (2007) 'Developing the commissioning strategy: From analysis to written document' in *Key Activities in Commissioning Adult Social Care*. London: CSIP.

HM Treasury (2003) *The Green Book: Appraisal and Evaluation in Central Government*. London: TSO. Available at: www.hm-treasury.gov.uk/data_greenbook_index.htm

Frontier Economics (2010) *Financial Benefits of Investment in Specialist Housing for Vulnerable and Older People*. London: HCA. Available at: www.education.gov.uk/research/data/uploadfiles/DFE-RR046.pdf; www.thesroinetwork.org/content/view/107/116/

Matrix Insight (2009) *Prioritising Investments in Preventative Health*. Health England.

6

Managing the Strategy and Communicating with Stakeholders

This chapter presents a further range of practical tools and activities to help commissioners develop and implement a commissioning strategy. In particular, it will describe tools which facilitate project, planning and communication.

Scenarios and case studies are presented to illustrate how commissioners from varying organisations have used the tools to commission for populations with specific needs.

Through stop and reflect activities, you will be encouraged to consider how you might make practical use of the ideas and tools discussed.

Learning outcomes

By the end of this chapter the reader should be able to:

- Understand and apply planning tools, such as project/review plans and gap analysis activity.
- Understand and apply communication tools, such as communications plans, commissioning intentions statements and market position statements.

Key terms

- *Critical path analysis* – a critical path analysis is a diagram showing what needs to be done and when.
- *Gantt chart* – a timeline that shows the progress of the different project activities and related costs.
- *Gap analysis* – a tool that helps evaluate the current position in relation to desired outcomes.
- *Market position statement* – a market-facing document bringing together data from joint strategic needs assessment, commissioning strategies, and market or customer surveys into a single document to inform and be of benefit to the provider sector.
- *Commissioning intentions statement* – a high level statement describing the direction of travel in commissioning services to deliver outcomes for a particular population. It acts as a 'marker' or signal to partners and providers.

Planning tools

Project planning

The development of commissioning strategies is best led by senior managers who should be well placed to mobilise and coordinate human and other resources from across the organisation. In doing so, a project management approach can prove helpful.

The IPC approach to project planning has seven stages:

- Agree the specification or terms of reference for the project.
- Plan the project, identifying roles and responsibilities, timescales, activities and resources.
- Communicate the plan to top team members and other stakeholders.
- Agree and delegate tasks.
- Manage and motivate the team.
- Monitor and review progress, modifying the plan and/or taking remedial action if necessary.
- Complete and publish the project.

Developing a commissioning strategy is a complex 'project' or process, with a range of interested stakeholders. When identifying the different roles and responsibilities you should consider having:

- A project sponsor to 'own' and back the project.
- A project steering group to oversee the development and review of the commissioning strategy.
- A project team (task and finish group) to undertake the necessary work on strategy development, analysis, procurement, implementation and monitoring.
- Project reference groups of provider agencies and other stakeholders, who would be responsible for testing, challenging and adding quality to the analysis.

Stop and Reflect

- How does this approach compare with the approach to project management in your organisation?
- What would be the main challenges to using this methodology in your organisation?

Critical path analysis

A critical path analysis can help manage complex projects. It shows project activities in a linear flow chart which is set against a timescale. It is particularly useful for showing where activities overlap or are interdependent.

Figure 6.1 shows a simplified critical path analysis for baking a cake. We start by collecting and preparing the necessary equipment and ingredients. The ingredients are combined in a particular order and placed in a baking tin. While this takes place the oven is warming. Some activities are dependent on the completion of earlier tasks, for example, the cake must be cooked before it can be iced.

Essentially, a critical path analysis is a diagram showing what needs to be done and when.

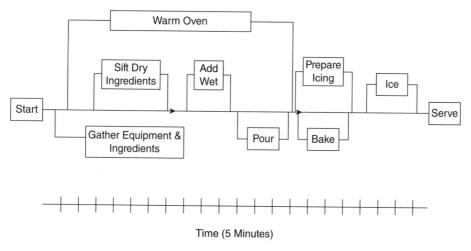

Time (5 Minutes)

Figure 6.1 A critical path analysis for baking a cake

Gantt chart

A Gantt chart is a timeline that shows the progress of the different project activities and related costs. They can be generated using a spreadsheet. Different colours are often used to show different types of project activity, such as stakeholder engagement/consultation. This tool is less effective in showing interdependencies than the critical path analysis but offers more scope for capturing costs and risks.

Activity	Time (5 minutes)	Costs (revenue)	Costs (capital)
Gathering ingredients & equipment		4	5
Warm oven		3	
Sift dry ingredients		3	2
Stir in wet ingredients		3	2
Pour into baking tin		2	
Cook		6	
Prepare icing		3	2
Ice cake		4	
Serve		3	
Total costs		31	11

Figure 6.2 A Gantt chart for baking a cake

Stop and Reflect

- How could you use a project management approach and tools to plan, deliver and monitor a commissioning strategy?

Monitoring and review plan

It is useful to decide at an early stage how the implementation of the strategy will be monitored and reviewed. A plan for monitoring and review might include:

- A set of measures or indicators which will allow the commissioners to monitor activity, performance and impact of the services commissioned.
- A framework which ensures that regular review meetings are held to analyse progress against commissioning objectives using the measures identified above, consider changes in the environment, and agree any changes to objectives or action plans or resources.
- A format which allows the opportunity for commissioners, providers and other stakeholders to contribute to the analysis of progress.
- Contracts, service level agreements and grants with providers that ensure they will collect the service activity and performance data necessary to enable effective monitoring to take place.

The monitoring and review plan will address the following questions:

- How are services performing against the agreed specification?
- Are services meeting assessed need?

- Are services being provided to the required standard?
- How much do they cost and are they providing value for money?
- Are appropriate services being commissioned?
- To what extent are services meeting commissioning objectives?
- What are the views of service providers, citizens, stakeholders and the wider public about the effectiveness of services?
- Are outcomes being achieved? Set measurable outcomes for citizens.

It will also pose questions about the effectiveness of the strategy itself, such as:

- Are the gaps in service need being met?
- Do commissioning priorities need to be changed?
- Do services need to be commissioned differently?
- Is there a need to review and reconfigure existing services?

Stop and Reflect

- Can you think of any examples from your own work where commissioning priorities have been changed as a result of review activities?

Communication tools

Communications plan

In developing a commissioning strategy, commissioners need to manage a complex set of relationships with partners, providers and service users. It is important, therefore, that commissioners demonstrate openness and fairness in relation to all stakeholders. A communications plan can help ensure transparency. It also helps to develop a common understanding of the commissioning process.

A communications plan should include:

- Written information – widely available information for all interested parties about the project and its findings as they develop. The written information might include a short briefing paper describing the project, its timetable and opportunities for stakeholders to contribute, and be followed by regular updates summarising key findings from each stage of the work.
- Interactive events – seminars and workshops for stakeholders at which findings from each stage of the project are presented and discussed, and where stakeholders have the opportunity to challenge and develop ideas.
- Formal research activities – such as interviews, focus groups, information and data collection from stakeholders as part of the methodology of the project.
- Formal decision making, including how the strategy will be presented.

Examples of comments from commissioners about the importance of communications plans are listed below:

> 'You need to carry out a full stakeholder analysis at the beginning, and ensure this considers internal stakeholders as well as external ones.'

> 'We set up a generic email address which was well publicised and available for anyone to use to make comments on plans.'

> 'Although there was political engagement in the process, and the political decision had been taken to close this particular day service, there were difficulties when the local members encountered local opposition ... it was important to maintain regular member briefings, particularly when it looked like the process could raise issues.'

> 'It was very important that our plan was translated into an accessible format and was presented in both Welsh and English.'

Commissioning intentions statement

This is a high level statement describing the direction of travel in commissioning services to deliver outcomes for particular populations. It acts as a 'marker' or signal to partners/providers so that any potential provider can understand the commissioner's approach to delivering outcomes for specific communities and populations.

A commissioning intentions statement may typically be structured into four sections:

- Outline of the commissioner's approach to commissioning and service delivery
- An explanation of the commissioner's commissioning framework
- Presentation of commissioning intentions
- Implications of the approach, including how the commissioner will approach decommissioning

---

Stop and Reflect

- How do you communicate and engage stakeholders in your organisation?
- How could you use these particular communication tools in your organisation?

Market position statement

Successive governments have emphasised ideas of choice and control for the users of social care. Consequently local authorities have less responsibility for providing services and more responsibility for creating a diverse social care market. For example:

> Social care already involves a diverse range of providers, including the voluntary and private sectors. But more can be done to make a reality of our vision of a thriving social market in which innovation flourishes. Councils have a role in stimulating, managing and shaping this market, supporting communities, voluntary organisations, social enterprises and mutual's to flourish and develop innovative and creative ways of addressing care needs. ... To build on this they will need robust evidence about what local markets offer and how they operate. (Department of Health, 2010: Para. 5.2)

Facilitation of the social care market requires local authorities to engage in three distinct tasks, as Figure 6.3 illustrates, and is discussed in detail in Chapter 8. Market intelligence involves a common and shared perspective of supply and demand, leading to an evidenced, published, market position statement for a given market. Market structuring involves the activities designed to give the market shape and structure, where commissioner behaviour is visible and the outcomes they are trying to achieve agreed, or at least accepted. Market intervention consists of the interventions commissioners make in order to deliver the kind of market believed to be necessary for any given community.

This section explores the first of these activities: the understanding of market intelligence through the development of market position statements.

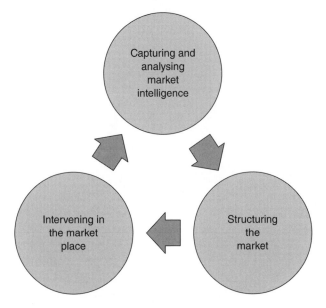

Figure 6.3 A model for understanding market facilitation

Developing market intelligence

To develop market intelligence, information needs to be gathered from three perspectives: what local authorities need to know, what providers need to know and what service users need to know.

The following are examples of questions that may help to gather market information from the three perspectives.

WHAT DOES THE LOCAL AUTHORITY NEED TO KNOW?

- Who provides what, where and at what price?
- What is the perceived quality of services provided?
- What is the relationship between activity, outcome and cost?
- What are the financial and business challenges facing different services and what are the key factors influencing success and viability?
- What do providers know about demand and how can this information best be used?
- What does an overall model of good practice look like and what would it cost to achieve? How close/far away is existing provision from that model?
- What are the key drivers behind demand and how can these be stopped, lessened or deferred?
- What are people saying about current services and their priorities for the future and what approaches are successful in enabling people with support needs to drive changes in the market?

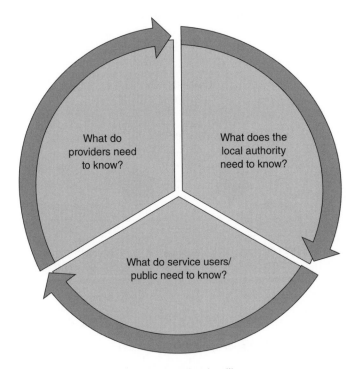

Figure 6.4   Information needed to gather market intelligence

What do service users/the public need to know?

- Who provides what, where and at what price?
- Are there good reviews (from a number of sources including other users) of the quality of service provision and does this have a strong user input?
- How can I get involved to ensure that the services that are available locally meet my aspirations for the future?
- What is meant by choice and control – and what choices might I have available to me in terms of choice of service, delivery or worker?
- What choices have other people made and how successful have they been in meeting their outcomes (including direct feedback from other users)?
- How flexible is the service I am being offered and does it remain under my control regardless of the purchase/payment mechanism?
- If you are a carer at the start of a caring role, what degree and what flexibility of support will be available to you?
- Do I have enough money (either from my own pocket or via my council's personal budget) to buy the type of care I need, and what other personal or community resources might I need to draw upon?

What do providers need to know?

- What does future demand look like and how reliable is this projection?
- What is the future balance of the market likely to be between self-funders, personal budget holders and those where the local authority intervenes more directly?
- What is the expected pace and scope of personal budget implementation and what impact will this have on the market?
- What are people (consumers) saying about current services and their aspirations for the future?
- Will there be consistency by the local authority towards price and support? What will the attitude be to transaction costs?
- Will the local authority be clear about what it considers to be a reasonable margin of profit?
- What will the attitude of planning authorities be to the development of new care facilities?
- Will the local authority support or incentivise innovation, and at what price?
- Does the local authority plan changes in its tendering processes or specification requirements that will promote or support change?
- Will the local authority incentivise diversification or start-up, for example through training, secondment of personnel, or provision of back office services?
- Will the local authority incentivise quality, how, and at what price?

Stop and Reflect

- From your perspective as a commissioner/service user/provider, would these questions provide all the information you require? Can you think of any other questions you would want answered?

Developing a market position statement

Once information has been gathered from a range of sources, a market position statement (MPS) is written. It draws together data from the joint strategic needs assessment (JSNA), commissioning strategies, and market and customer surveys into a single document.

The market position statement should be market facing, that is, contain information the authority believes, and can substantiate, would be of benefit to care providers.

As Figure 6.5 illustrates, an MPS is not a repetition of a JSNA or a commissioning strategy but a practical document that is focused on delivering a specific product to benefit the market.

Local Authority Strategic Planning

JSNA	Commissioning Strategy	Market Position Statement
Defines demand across health, housing and social care. Essentially a broad-based statement of current and future trends.	Normally based around groups of service users, commissioning strategies should:	An analytical, 'market facing' document that brings together material from the JSNA and commissioning strategies into a document that presents the data the market needs to know if they are to plan their future role and function.
May help to identify and target key populations, using predictive risk modelling.	Build on the view of demand presented by the JSNA. Identify current practice and future use of public resources.	Identifies the needs and preferences of different service user groups in the market, e.g. older people, learning disability, etc. and covers local authority and privately funded users of care.
Looks at long term patterns of need and demand.	Look at the resources the local authority has available and how these may be allocated or re-allocated in the future.	Indicates the necessary changes, characteristics and innovation to service design and delivery the local authority would like to see in the market to meet the needs and preferences of the whole population, and how the local authority will support and intervene in local markets.

Figure 6.5 Comparative characteristics of a JSNA, commissioning strategy and MPS

In addition a market position statement should:

- Cover the whole provider market, not just that part which the local authority currently funds.
- Indicate how the local authority intends to behave towards the market in the future.
- Be a brief and analytical rather than descriptive document.
- Be evidence-informed, in that each statement it makes has a rationale that underpins it, based on population estimates, market surveys, research and so on.
- Take into account and (as relevant to the user group) consider the role of the wider local authority; for example, housing, education, leisure services and health services.

A market position statement is an important tool in starting constructive and creative dialogue between the local authority and its public, private and voluntary sector providers.

So what should a market position statement contain? A potential outline is described below:

- *A summary of the direction the local authority and its partners wish to take and the purpose of the document*: A summary of the key care and wellbeing objectives for the local community; the principles of policy, legislation and regulation that will have an impact on the market; a summary of the key elements of the analysis presented in the individual sections below.
- *The local authority's predictions of future demand, identifying key pressure points*: An analysis of the current population and anticipated projections for the coming 5, 10 and 15 years for the relevant market sector and the impact any population change may have on future demand for health, housing and care services; an analysis concerned with the whole care and wellbeing market, including for example, self-funders and those funded by the local authority either in part or in total. Consumer perspectives should be represented in here; an evaluation of particular aspects of demand now and in the future, for example, by geography (which wards have high density) and by nature of particular problems, for example, dementia, profound and multiple disabilities. This will include the rationale on which such estimates are being made. It includes aspects of service demand that might reduce.
- *The local authority's view of the current state of supply covering both strengths and weaknesses within the market*: A review of current spend and by whom on particular market sectors; a quantitative picture of current supply, looking at what services are provided, to whom, where and in what volume; a qualitative picture of current supply indicating those areas where services appear not to be meeting required standards or users' requirements or outcomes. This might include summaries of CQC reports, of complaints, of user surveys and mystery shopper exercises.
- *Identified models of practice the local authority and its partners will encourage*: A review of how the local authority sees the supply side delivering in the future in terms of the approaches and methodologies that might be used; an analysis of the extent to which desired models of care are matched by current provision, and whether they would require increased funding to deliver a different approach; suggestions as to how might the market deliver change; a statement about whether the local authority will continue to provide or directly purchase any services, whether it will seek framework agreements with providers or seek only to influence CQC, service users, carers, government in particular directions.
- *The likely future level of resourcing*: Which areas of supply the LA will see as a high priority, where it wishes to see services develop and those areas where it would be less likely to purchase or encourage service users to purchase in the future; a description of the vision and options for future resourcing, and how this matches with the shift in resources that may be desired by the previous section; if cuts are to be made an analysis of the likely targets, an analysis of the services which might be de-commissioned or discouraged and how will the LA seek to achieve changes.
- *The support the LA will offer towards providing choice as well as innovation and development*: An analysis of what the authority anticipates will be the impact of more service

users purchasing or negotiating their own care, and what impact might this have on transaction costs; any particular offers available to providers, for example, outcome-based contracts, land availability, help with planning consent, guaranteed or underwritten take up of services, training and development, business and management support, if they develop certain types of provision.

Stop and Reflect

- Do you have examples of market position statements in your local authority?
- How effective is it/are they in developing a dialogue with providers about supply, demand and the possible design of future services?

CASE STUDY

As a result of national and local drivers, Borsetshire Council decided to move from a model of traditional domiciliary care and housing related support to an outcome-based approach. Working in partnership with Health Service colleagues, Borsetshire ran a series of consultative workshops with service users and carers. The workshops generated some key messages from service users; for example:

- I want help when I am in a crisis
- I want to be free from abuse
- I want you to be honest with me
- I want to stay at home as long as possible
- I want to feel safe
- I want to speak to someone face to face
- I want good quality information that is easy to access
- I want to be able to go to the toilet independently
- I want to see and talk to people
- I want to know what it will cost me

The feedback from service users helped Borsetshire Council to identify the gaps or weaknesses in current provision:

- They needed to improve their information and advice to both people who might fund their own care as well as their own 'customers'.
- They needed to look carefully at how they responded to older people when they were in a crisis (and not to rush to make a long-term decision for someone at the time of the crisis).
- They needed to ensure that their staff were clear about the options that people who came to them for help faced and that there were services in place to address whatever the presenting needs were.

- Most of all they wanted to create a more holistic response which focused on helping older people remain in their own homes or their own communities.

As a result of this analysis the council's commissioners began to design possible service delivery models. At this stage the commissioners also began to engage providers in conversation so they could understand the implications of service redesign from a provider perspective.

The final outcome of this work was a redesigned service specification and model of service delivery.

Summary

In this chapter, project planning and communication tools which support the implementation of a commissioning strategy have been presented and explained.

An approach to project planning was described, including the use of critical path analysis and Gantt charts.

Three particular tools or methodologies were included in the section on communication: an approach to planning effective communication; an example of a commission intentions statement, and a discussion of the purpose and an approach to developing a market position statement.

References

Learning and Skills Council (North East) Regional Commissioning Statement (2010), Feb. Gateshead: LSC.

Department of Health (2010) *A Vision for Adult Social Care: Capable communities and active citizens*. London: Department of Health.

7

Towards Effective Service Design

Service design is a key element of the commissioning process for commissioners, providers and service users. It requires thought and time to: involve stakeholders, engage staff, develop plans, identify resources, and implement a new or redesigned service.

This chapter looks at what is meant by service design and presents a range of approaches and some tools to help you do it. It identifies some key principles, the different phases or stages of the service design process, and the activities required. There is no one ideal way to design services effectively, but it is hoped that this chapter will equip you to decide on the approach that best suits the context in which you are working.

At the time of writing, there is an expectation of greater integration of health and social care services as a means of improving: the service user's experience, reducing duplication, and pooling resources in a constrained financial environment. For this to succeed, careful consideration is needed as to how best to design services with partners or other organisations in a way that builds stakeholder engagement from the very start of the process. This chapter covers the issues that may confront you in designing services with partners and other organisations.

Learning outcomes

By the end of this chapter you should be able to:

- Understand the concept of service design.
- Recognise different approaches to, and tools for, service design.
- Identify potential barriers and enabling factors to good service design.

What is service design and redesign?

Service design can be defined as the activity of planning and organising people, infrastructure, communication and the components of a service, in order to improve quality, the interaction between the service provider and customers, and the customer's experience.

Effective service design in public care provides an opportunity for commissioners and providers to maximise existing resources, bring new resources into the equation, involve stakeholders and minimise costs. It involves:

- Analysing existing arrangements
- Identifying gaps, overlaps and duplication
- Consideration of costs, pathways and staffing
- Taking account of culture and the agreed benefits of the change

There is a tendency for organisations to continue with historic arrangements for service provision, with small incremental changes over time. Radical change is rarer and often more difficult to implement. However, financial constraints and greater pressure for efficiencies in recent years have forced many local authorities to review their services, and provided a new urgency to identifying what services to commission and how best they can be delivered.

Growing interest in co-production where service users work with providers to design and deliver services has also developed in parallel with the financial constraints on public sector budgets. Co-production means:

> delivering public services in an equal and reciprocal relationship between professionals, people using services, their families and their neighbours. Where activities are co-produced in this way, both services and neighbourhoods become far more effective agents of change. (Boyle and Harris, 2009)

One evaluation study cited by Bubb (2012), found that 49% of local authorities reported cost benefits as a result of involving parents in commissioning and shaping services.

Taking a service design approach which means looking at how services may best achieve strategic objectives, and helps to think afresh about what services are needed and how they could best be delivered. This approach may help both commissioners and providers to ensure that services are effectively designed to meet the needs of clients.

Types of change in service redesign

When looking at designing or redesigning a service, possible changes tend to fall into seven areas:

- Change in location, e.g. respite at home instead of respite centre.
- Change in the method of delivery, e.g. from face to face to telephone service or assistive technology.
- Substituting skills, e.g. multi-disciplinary team instead of health or social care specialists.
- Supporting co-production, e.g. self-assessment, direct payments.
- Simplifying access or pathways, e.g. self-assessment and referral to community equipment services.
- Targeting, e.g. falls services targeted at those most at risk of falling.
- Integration of services, e.g. reablement services, learning disability services.

These are not mutually exclusive: for example, the introduction of a reablement service might involve changes across all seven areas as a new integrated service might involve a change in location and method of delivery, provided by a team of specially trained staff from across health and social care, targeted at those most likely to benefit with a strong ethos of enablement, and involving a simplified referral and assessment process.

Approaches to service design and redesign

In any service design exercise in public care, there are three possible approaches that are potentially useful to providers and commissioners of services:

- *Outcome-focused approaches* focusing on the impact of the service on an individual's quality of life and how it can help them to achieve their desired outcomes.
- *Pathways approaches* focusing on the individual's journey through the service and how to provide accessible and easy to use services with a clear pathway from beginning to end from the individual's perspective.
- *Whole systems approaches* which cut across professional disciplines and organisational boundaries, potentially pooling resources and reducing duplication to provide seamless care for individuals.

Some degree of person-centredness is embedded in each of these three approaches. This contrasts with traditional approaches to service design where content and/or forms of delivery are standardised, or are determined solely by those who deliver them. Designing services in the traditional way may offer little opportunity for creativity, innovation or service user involvement.

Outcome-focused approaches

Outcome-focused approaches require fundamental change in the way that services are delivered. Outcome-based approaches are about changing:

> the social care system away from the traditional service provision with its emphasis on inputs and processes towards a more flexible, efficient approach, which delivers the outcomes people want and need and promotes their independence, well-being and dignity. (Department of Health, 2008b)

This means, for example, that if you are looking at a day centre service you stand back and review with stakeholders what the outcomes are that this service is aiming to achieve. This might mean, for example, replacing day centre sessions with support and the opportunity to take part in a canal boat restoration project – helping to achieve the outcomes of reduced social isolation and increased confidence.

Using an outcome-focused approach to design services will mean a different role for providers and commissioners: offering providers greater responsibility for designing services to achieve the outcomes identified by service users and commissioners; while commissioners focus on identifying, specifying and monitoring outcomes. A focus on outcomes enables providers to work more creatively and flexibly with service users in designing services to meet service users' desired outcomes. Thus, it may result in different services and gives service users greater choice and control, focusing on their capacities and aspirations rather than deficits.

A Council decided to design a 'Help to Live at Home Service' composed of the domicilliary care service, an integrated equipment and telecare service, and an out of hours response service. The service was to be built around the wishes of service users and expressed in relation to those outcomes they wanted that would help them move towards greater independence.

They held a number of events, with local NHS Trusts as partners, where they invited professionals and older people to work together in looking to create a better care pathway for people who may require services. They held workshops across the county at which at least 20% of those involved were carers or users of services. Alongside these

CASE STUDY

(Continued)

(Continued)

events it undertook an extensive consultation with existing and potential customers and their carers.

The messages from the consultation confirmed what was really important for older people in their care services. The Council began to focus its thinking in a number of directions but critically saw weaknesses in its own current arrangements:

- They needed to improve their information and advice to both people who might fund their own care as well as their own 'customers'.
- They needed to look carefully at how they responded to older people when they were in a crisis (and not to rush to make a long-term decision for someone at the time of the crisis).
- They needed to ensure that their staff were clear about the options that people who came to them for help faced and that there were services in place to address whatever the presenting needs were.
- Most of all they wanted to create a more holistic response which focused on helping older people remain in their own homes or their own communities.

They began thinking of making reablement not just a six-week process but the basis on which all services were commissioned and provided.

The Council constructed a first draft of their service specification for a new outcome-based service in which there was no limit to the period of recovery/reablement. Alongside this process of looking at how to procure services, was a growing recognition that many of the ways in which older people's care and support needs might be met did not rest in the traditional services that might be provided or commissioned by the Council, but would be found with older people in their communities.

As a consequence, the whole basis of the contractual relationship with providers is changed. The provider is now allocated a sum of money based on the defined outcomes that the older person and their assessment and care management worker have agreed. The provider is then responsible with the customer for the delivery of those outcomes. The service can be described as 'personalised', in that it offers an individually tailored package according to the outcomes agreed and specified by the customer.

Monitoring outcome-focused services

There are considerable challenges in identifying measurable outcomes against which to measure success. Glendinning et al. (2006) classify outcomes in terms of change, maintenance and process outcomes. While change outcomes are relatively easy to measure – for example, supporting someone with mental health problems into employment – maintenance and process outcomes may be more difficult and more time-consuming to measure and monitor – for example, maintaining independent living and providing a service that respects the dignity of the service user. A number of tools have been developed which can be used by providers to identify, evaluate and monitor outcomes. These include:

ASCOT – Adult Social Care Outcomes Toolkit which is used to measure improvement in outcomes for individuals and can measure: changes over time; current and expected situation in the absences of a service; expected gain from service use; and capacity of the individuals to benefit from a service (Netten et al., 2011).

Talking Points (Scotland) – is an approach which is seen to provide an opportunity to 'get back to basics' in working with individuals and families to identify the goals they want to achieve. Talking Points provides a framework for commissioners or those involved in commissioning to use in order to get people talking about the outcomes they want to achieve during assessment and support planning processes (Cook and Miller, 2012).

Outcomes Star – is a scoring system measuring wellbeing on a number of areas which are relevant to the individual. Further information is available at: www.outcomesstar.org.uk/

An outcomes-focused approach to service design is allied to outcome-focused service specifications. These give providers the opportunity to work with service users on the more detailed design of a service.

CASE STUDY

A Borough Council Extra Care and Support scheme provides a mixture of approximately 240 tenure options and support arrangements to approximately 50 clients funded by the Borough Council Child and Adult Services. The care and support to the Council-funded clients has been designed and delivered according to an outcome based specification and a care and support planning template.

There were three outcomes specified in the contract:

- Contribute to the initial reduction of the levels of care and/or support previously received by the service user before entering the scheme.
- Support the on-going care and support needs of its service users and reduce the likelihood of admission to long term care.
- Contribute to the prevention of hospital admission, re-admission and enable early discharge.

In addition to the three outcomes specified above, the provider was also required to deliver health promotion outcomes to both service users and residents of the wider community. Examples of individual outcomes that the service will need to deliver include:

- Contribute to supporting people to live independently, remain healthier and recover more quickly from illness or accident.
- Contribute to improving the independence and quality of life of people with long term conditions. Assist people in developing and maintaining a positive, active and productive approach to their lives.

Pathways approach

An alternative approach to service design or redesign is the pathways approach, based on the concept of the service user following a pathway or journey through part of the public care system. The concept of 'service journeys' was pioneered and trialled in Scandinavia. The approach is increasingly being applied to services in the public and private sectors as it enables people to see how experiences of service use play out in reality. The focus is not so much on understanding and optimising operational processes, but on developing the best experience for service users.

The pathway approach can involve thinking about a hypothetical service user and how they would access and navigate the proposed service, or looking at the pathway of current service users. By mapping the pathway it is possible to identify potential pinch points along the pathway where additional resources are needed and to think about the wider implications of a change in service for other staff and organisations. For example, in planning an integrated discharge service, mapping the pathway from admission to six weeks post discharge of a hypothetical older person may highlight the need to plan for:

- The recruitment of additional staff in the community
- New IT systems to track people along the pathway
- Training a variety of health, social care and housing staff in new procedures and protocols

Mapping service user pathways and understanding the route people take into, through and out of services, can help in the alignment of provision. It can also help to identify which elements of a service are amenable to integration and the areas which need to be addressed, such as information sharing and the skills and expertise needed to support the user. Examining the referrals process and looking at ways of improving initial assessments can often help to target resources more effectively by ensuring the right support is provided at the right point in time. In defining pathways it is important that service designers listen to the experience of service users. Well conducted consultations will uncover areas of duplication in provision, and equally, areas of fragmentation where a service is poor because one element does not know what the other is delivering.

A pathways approach will require providers and commissioners to address: staffing and skills, roles and responsibilities, process and timing issues, location and outcomes. There is a greater emphasis when using this approach on the process and the service user's experience along the pathway compared with the focus on the end result of the outcome-based approach.

Whole-system approach

A third approach to service design is to take a whole-system perspective. This means thinking about the whole system that contributes to the health and wellbeing of a person, and leads to identification of a range of key areas which may need to be addressed in designing or redesigning it. For example, in designing a service for people with mental health needs, a whole system approach may highlight resources and budgets available across social care, mental health, criminal justice, leisure services, housing etc. It will require consideration of: IT services; the organisational cultures involved and any development needs; the available workforce across the system and training needs. This approach may also help to identify avoidable duplication of services across the system.

An example of a whole-system approach to service design is the Total Place initiative (2010) in England. This involved 13 pilots covering a combined population of 13 million people, 63 local authorities, 34 Primary Care Trusts, 12 fire authorities, 13 police authorities, and a wide range of third sector organisations and service delivery bodies. The pilots demonstrated service improvements and savings. The key elements of the approach were defined as:

- Starting from the citizen viewpoint to break down the organisational and service silos which cause confusion to citizens, create wasteful burdens of data collection and management on the frontline, and which contribute to poor alignment of services; and
- Providing strong local, collective and focused leadership which supports joined up working and shared solutions to problems with citizens at the heart of service design.

The whole-system approach is particularly useful in shifting focus from the specific service to its wider context, and the other services and activities that may be relevant to the service user. This can help to identify additional resources in situations where one person or group may be receiving a range of fragmented and uncoordinated services. However, the challenge may be to unlock these resources from their various silos in order to provide a single more effective service as organisations or departments often resist pooling resources.

Service design phases

The activities involved in effective service design, whether focused on outcomes, pathways or whole sysytems, may be broken down into four phases:

- Pre-design.
- Design.
- Testing.
- Implementation.

Monitoring and review may then lead to further design or redesign in a continuous circle of service design.

Pre-design phase

The purpose of this phase is to produce agreement on the design principles and outcomes for the model of service. These principles should be fundamental statements about what you are trying to achieve and about your approach. For example, the principles underpinning and influencing the design of a brokerage service could be: 'We will put in place access to a range of brokerage support planning that allows the individual together with whoever provides the care and support required to determine what needs to be offered, when and how, in order to achieve the outcomes desired by the individual.' And in terms of the approach: 'Change will be managed by those most affected.'

At this stage, in thinking about the design, it will be helpful to:

- Focus on high level redesign (keep the detail for the implementation stage).
- Concentrate on what the new process will be, not how it will be introduced.
- Identify the work which needs to be done (tasks), not who will do them.
- Reduce the number of 'process steps' to a minimum.
- Describe the 'natural order' of processes and tasks.
- Ensure that as many tasks as possible are performed in the same team or location.
- Perform work where it makes sense, not necessarily where it happens now.
- Support the smooth running of the process with protocols and guidelines.
- Design jobs which deliver the process, not protect the status quo.
- Empower staff to make decisions about the process.
- Build in review and monitoring.
- Identify both financial, staffing, IT and time constraints.

This is also the point at which to identify who are the stakeholders and to think about how they are going to be involved. It will be important for those involved on a day to day basis to understand the overall vision, commissioning intentions or outcomes that are required to be delivered. The project team will need skills in change and project management, influencing and engagement.

Stop and Reflect

These are some questions you may find helpful to ask at the pre-design stage:

- What are the boundaries of the service design?
- What is the redesign issue?
- What are the elements of the system?
- What will be your approach? Is this going to be a radical redesign of the organisation's processes, or an incremental, continuous approach to change?
- What is your justification for the focus on these areas?
- What information do you need to be clear about the issue and to help you decide what needs to be done to address the issue?
- Can you learn from experience of previous changes?
- What do you need to do differently?
- What other national and local change agendas, corporate initiatives or programmes need to complement this agenda?

- Who are the key stakeholders inside and outside the organisation?
- How can you engage them and build support and consensus?
- What arrangements are needed to enable stakeholders to work together?
- Are there incentives or benefits for those affected?

Design phase

The aim of the design phase is to develop the outline design of the service or Target Operating Model (TOM). A TOM can only be developed once the organisation has clarity and agreement about its service vision.

The TOM describes the high level view of the individual constituent parts of the whole system that is required to deliver the vision. It also identifies a number of key design principles and characteristics that will inform the more detailed work required to develop the actual model. At a minimum it should include: the function of the new/redesigned service; the future internal structures; who is involved; the processes and external service developments required for the organisation to take it forward; and a clear statement of how it will link with other parts of the organisation.

TOM components typically include:

- Vision
- Function of service
- Who does what?
- Supporting documents and processes
- Additional activities
- Pictorial models

The development of a TOM does not mean that a 'perfect design' has been achieved – it has merely pointed the organisation in a certain direction for further exploration. Work will continue to be undertaken on understanding the impacts of that direction and design, and the capacity and skill needed within the organisation to manage the changes effectively.

This is very much a 'top down' approach to service design and redesign, and may lead to poorer performance and a worsened care experience if not done thoroughly. The concept of a TOM should be seen as a blueprint as opposed to a fixed design. Typically the final design of the new approach can be influenced by the option to:

- Make a series of modifications to the existing service/process model to meet the design principles identified in the previous stage, or
- Explore an already existing model or design used elsewhere, for example the In-Control seven stage process for service users, or
- Develop on a 'blank page' – a completely new and unique solution to meet the design principles.

Services should not be shoe-horned into a TOM if it is clear that this will not meet the objectives of the organisation. For example, if the objective is to improve customer access and the model does not do this, then it is not the correct model.

Stop and Reflect

These are some questions you may find helpful at the design stage:

- What approaches are available to tackle this issue?
- Does the design impact in areas where there are currently high costs – for instance, contributing to avoiding a hospital admission or reducing the period of intensive service provision?
- Will the change or new service design contribute to improving early detection or improve early intervention and minimise the demand for more intensive services in the future?
- Which approaches that fit with current service provision are likely to be most successful?
- Are there similar successful examples elsewhere: why did they work in these areas; would they work in your own authority?
- You may identify issues that are important or high cost with a big impact – but will they face opposition and resistance from staff, service users and carers or potential providers?
- What is the balance of the cost of the change and ongoing costs against the value of benefits?
- Are there significant changes to the resources needed to fund these changes?
- How will you begin to bring the design together?
- What approaches, project tools or other systems may help?
- Can you 'test it' through scenario testing, role play, or piloting to find out if the model will meet the needs of service users?
- What will a good design look like? How big a difference will it make?
- What could possibly happen to affect the project? (For example, outside influences such as changes in funding.)
- How will you ensure effective communication and engagement across key partners and stakeholders including users and carers?
- What skills are needed within the organisation to ensure effective project and risk management?

Testing phase

The purpose of this phase is to find out if the model will meet the needs of service users and to help predict and prevent problems.

Having developed a workable design, some organisations will introduce a new service without fully testing the new arrangements. There may be very good reasons to do this, but some form of testing should be considered when:

- The scope of the new design is large or complex.
- The new model/service could cause far-reaching, unintended consequences.
- Implementing the design and/or solutions will be a costly process.
- The design and/or solutions would be difficult to reverse.

You should consider the advantages of running a new service as a pilot in order to:

- Understand the resources realistically required to run the model or service.
- Understand the true performance of the system or model.
- Identify additional improvements.
- Understand and improve how the new design can be fully implemented effectively.
- Provide opportunities to engage with users and stakeholders on the new arrangements.

If difficulties and problems arise during the pilot, it is quite likely that they would have occurred at the time of implementation. This initial phase gives you a chance to identify and address them before they become widely applied.

Scenario testing

To ensure that a service design will actually meet the needs of service users and will not have unintended negative consequences on the overall whole system, scenario testing can help you to predict and prevent problems. A well designed exercise can be valuable where it allows participants to work through how a new service might work, and to consider the dangers of any unintended consequences of new arrangements. It can help all stakeholders test the feasibility of a proposed service development, as well as identify additional guidance, protocols or arrangements needed to make the service work well.

There are a number of approaches to service modelling and scenario testing, essentially based around the idea of a game which models the scenarios likely to prevail in real life if a particular service were to be introduced. They can vary from the basic and simple – for example, desk-based activities looking at the financial implications of changes to services, to more complicated exercises – such as role-playing activities involving dozens of actors more or less successfully acting out what they imagine would be the behaviour of different stakeholders in a particular new scenario. They can often involve following service users through the proposed service model. It can help all stakeholders to test the feasibility of a proposed service development, as well as identify additional guidance, protocols or arrangements needed to ensure the service works well.

Consensus of benefits

It is possible that some stakeholders will resist changes to existing or new services and therefore prior to implementation of any service design or redesign, it is useful to try to ensure that everyone is happy with the new design as this will facilitate implementation. If you have followed good practice in the process of designing the service, having established a strong rationale for the change and how it will improve service quality, it should be clear that the benefits will outweigh the disadvantages. This will help you to develop and maintain stakeholder engagement during the implementation stage.

Implementation

Implementation is the last phase of service design. However, following implementation there is frequently a need for further adjustments to services as the new arrangements go live and operational issues emerge. In addition, when staff actually start to implement and deliver a new or redesigned service, there is scope for what Lipsky (1980) in a classic text called the 'street level bureaucrat' to bend the service in ways that may not have been foreseen at the design stage. So for example, the implementation of FACS criteria (which are used by local authorities to determine eligibility for social care) may vary according to the practices and perceptions of those charged with carrying out an assessment service.

Therefore, as these examples illustrate there is a need to monitor and review any new service in order to assess whether further changes in the design are required and so the circle of service design continues.

Principles of service design and redesign

Running through most approaches to service design and redesign are a number of principles: stakeholder involvement, communication, evidence-informed, and based on national and local priorities.

Stakeholder involvement

There has been a growing recognition of the importance of stakeholder involvement in service design. According to *Commissioning for Personalisation: A Framework for Local Authority Commissioners* (DH, 2008a), 'Enabling meaningful participation for citizens in the commissioning process through active co-design, co-production and co-delivery, rather than post facto consultation' is a key principle for personalised commissioning. The Framework continues:

> Key tasks for operational commissioning are: Engaging citizens in commissioning – by developing outlets and formal mechanisms for citizens to be actively involved in service design and priority setting – not just as feedback. This may cover both universal and specialist services that lie outside of personal budgets as well as those services that can be directly purchased by individuals.

Stakeholders can include: commissioners, providers, managers, workforce, partner organisations, service users, carers and the wider community. It is important that all those who have a stake in the service which is being designed or redesigned are involved early on in the design process. They all have a part to play in thinking about existing arrangements, identifying gaps, overlaps and duplication, and what needs to happen to achieve the outcomes which the service is intended to deliver.

Communication

Stakeholder involvement is strengthened through effective, regular communication. A successful service design process will aim throughout to maintain communication with all those concerned as a way of ensuring that people can feed into the process, are aware of timescales and deadlines, and understand what is being designed and the rationale behind it. Keeping people up-to-date with the progress of service design and listening to their views and suggestions helps to ensure that the final design or redesign is effective and meets individual needs. Communication planning needs to address a number of key questions about the: communicator, message, communication channel, feedback mechanism, target audience, and time frame.

Evidence base

The evidence base for what actually works is quite weak in primary health and social care, particularly around prevention. Although the body of research is growing, we still do not know much about the relative effectiveness, or the relative costs and benefits, of different care service designs. However, effective service design should be based, as far as possible, on the available evidence about what designs work best. For example, in recent years, a number of studies have demonstrated that parenting programmes are cost effective and provide benefits to parents and children (London Economics, 2007) resulting in the further development of these services through Surestart and other initiatives.

Local and national priorities

A key principle for effective service design is that it should be informed by national and local priorities. For example, many local authorities and NHS organisations have developed services to address the government's policy of promoting reablement services for older people, taking advantage of additional funding and tailored to local circumstances. Designing services that reflect national and local priorities may be necessary to meet statutory requirements and offer an opportunity to access additional funding. However, there is always a risk that national priorities will shift, which may leave a newly designed service underfunded or no longer required.

Tools for service design and redesign

There are a wide range of bespoke tools used by organisations across the public, private and voluntary care sectors to help support better service design. They can be useful to commisioners when working with their providers to effect service improvement and better outcomes.

Re-engineering or business process re-engineering (BPR)

Re-engineering has its origins in the private sector as a way of helping organisations examine and rework business processes to improve the quality and efficiency of production and improve the customer experience. It often involves radical redesign of an organisation's processes. 'We have always done it this way' does not apply! An example from the world of industry is the re-engineering of traditional car manufacturing where each process uses specialised skills to build the car before passing it to the next stage in the process. Each process deals with a small part of the product without communication with other processes. After re-engineering, a small team of specialised workers might deal with each car, one at a time. Narrow specialists have been replaced by multi-skilled workers, and specialist teams replaced by cross-functional teams.

BPR involves total disassociation from current practices, starting with a clean slate and looking at the organisation as a whole. Change is usually top-down, and it can therefore seem an autocratic and non-democratic process. It requires strong and inspiring leadership. There is a danger that it can lead to an over-emphasis on technology and efficiency, reflecting its origins in private industry. Some parts of the health and care system do lend themselves in particular to this kind of approach. In social care, the introduction of direct payments and self-directed support lend themselves to BPR where a radical policy change has required an examination and fundamental rethink of care planning and management processes (IDeA, 2006).

Total Quality Management (TQM)

In contrast to BPR, Total Quality Management is a tool that focuses on an incremental approach to service design and redesign. TQM is based on the assumption that services can always be improved and that the quality of products and processes is the responsibility of everyone involved in the creation or consumption of a service, including management, workforce and service users. All stakeholders regularly review and discuss ways to improve service quality.

While re-engineering involves radical change in design, TQM involves incremental and continuous improvement through a logical sequence of four activities:

- Plan – plan ahead for change
- Do – execute the plan in small steps
- Study – check the results
- Act – take action to standardise or improve

There are three important aspects of TQM:

- Counting – needs statistical thinking and tools and behaviours to solve problems.
- Customers – do it because it is the best and only way to meet customer needs.
- Culture – relies on bottom-up, participative decision making.

TQM owes its prominence to Japanese economic success and approaches to quality adopted by leading Japanese companies which were popularised by Deming and others from the 1980s on (DTI, 2005).

TQM can only be successful if an organisation's culture supports the concept, for example, cooperation rather than competition as the basis for working together, with employees feeling a sense of ownership in, or engagement with, the organisation's objectives. In public care where quality is a central goal, TQM offers a useful aid to service design and redesign (DTI, 2005).

Lean thinking

Lean thinking (like TQM) emerged from Japanese industrial practices and the improvements in productivity achieved by Toyota in car manufacture. The primary focus was to make cars in the quickest and most efficient way, and to deliver them as quickly as possible – thereby eliminating waste which comes in three forms: *Muri* which focuses on the preparation and planning of the process, or what work can be avoided proactively by design; *mura* which focuses on how the work design is implemented and the elimination of fluctuation at the scheduling or operations level, such as quality and volume; and *muda* which may be discovered after the process is in place and is seen through variation in output. There are seven types of *muda*: unnecessary transport of goods, inventory – not processing all the components, unnecessary motion of people, waiting for the next stage in the process, overproduction of the product (or service), over-processing the product, and defects (and the time spent fixing them).

When government departments are under pressure to improve services with fewer resources, many adopt lean approaches to services as a means of improving services while eliminating waste. This means designing services to ensure that the service user gets what they need, where they need it, when they need it, without waiting. It involves understanding the value of each step from the service users' perspective, and not doing things that add no value from their perspective.

Research has shown that lean thinking can be successfully applied to the public sector. Pilot implementation studies commissioned by the Scottish Executive in public sector organisations including local authorities and the NHS were investigated and reported improvements in customer waiting times, service performance, processing times, customer flow, quality, efficiencies and cost savings (Radnor et al., 2006). Less tangible benefits included: generating a better understanding of the process; more joined-up working; improved use of performance data; increased staff satisfaction and confidence; and embedding a continuous improvement culture.

Best Value

Best Value is a government initiative which requires local authorities to ensure services meet the needs of local people in terms of quality, competitiveness, efficiency, continuous improvement and accountability.

Best Value shares principles of TQM with its emphasis on:

- Customer focus: User consultation is key, involving the collection of views of a range of customers. There is an expectation that there will be a two-way communication process with a performance plan that channels information back to users on achievements and plans for improvement.
- Continuous improvement: Statistical data is regularly collected on service performance. A performance plan and action plan are expected to identify performance measures of service success, along with strategies for improvement.

Statutory guidance on Best Value in September 2011 (Communities and Local Government, 2011) sets out the expectations on local authority commissioners to: consider overall value, including economic, environmental and social value; consult (at all stages of the commissioning cycle); to be responsive to the benefits and needs of the voluntary and community sector (VCS) and small businesses; and to avoid passing on disproportionate reductions to VCS and small businesses.

Solutions to obstacles towards effective service design

If you are working as a commissioner on the design of services, a number of factors may determine how effective you will be:

- Rationale. Change for change sake can lead to 'change fatigue' and de-motivated staff. Creating enough sense of purpose and a clearly articulated reason for the change is essential. Moreover some changes may have 'unpleasant' consequences (e.g. redundancies, greater performance management) and being really clear at the start about what you want to achieve and why, is essential if you are to manage these issues.

- Leadership. Whether or not the approach is top-down or participative and bottom-up, leadership is important in engaging with stakeholders, building consensus, and maintaining high morale throughout the various phases of the design process. Service change needs a level of project management, analysis and leadership skills. It is not essential that one individual holds all of these skills and more, but that the team or group of people overseeing the programme develop or have these skills already. In addition, visible senior buy-in and support is important in order to give the new service the necessary status and emphasis that it needs across an organisation.
- Organisational culture. Some service designs will require a culture change in the organisation: for example, introducing a more enabling way of working with service users; or it could be about breaking down professional or organisational cultures to work in a more multi-disciplinary way, or to facilitate greater collaboration with other services. Cultural issues across organisations can make or break service change programmes. Changing people's values and beliefs is central to any major or significant redesign of services.
- Resources. Most service design or redesign will require additional resources – if only for the changeover period from the previous service to the new service. Additional resources for stakeholder engagement and communication, staff training and new technology, are also frequently required.
- IT. Ensuring that you have the technology in place to deliver service change is increasingly important. Where joint working or partnerships are involved, this may mean having data-sharing protocols in place, as well as compatible systems.
- Risk and sensitivity analysis. Tools for option appraisal, such as cost benefit analysis, include a stage for risk and sensitivity analysis in the methodology. This means identifying risks and their potential impact and taking steps to mitigate where possible while also exploring the consequences of changes in key elements of the service – for example, varying impact of different rates of inflation. A common concern is the unforeseen consequences of a new or redesigned service – for example the development of perverse incentives for staff or service users to act inefficiently.
- Performance measures, monitoring and review. Just as it is important to be clear about the objectives for a new or redesigned service, it is also necessary to develop and agree on how performance will be measured and monitored as part of the service design. You will need to build review into the service design with the scope for feedback to support and achieve further improvements in the service.

Stop and Reflect

There are some final questions to consider before your new or redesigned service goes live:

- How will you know that the service has achieved the objectives and outcomes? What are the success criteria?
- What information do you need to find out if the service is effective?
- What systems will you need to understand effectiveness of changes?

Summary

This chapter has introduced you to key concepts, principles and tools for the design of effective services in public care, including outcomes-focused, pathways and whole systems approaches. The chapter highlights the important of building stakeholder involvement and communication into any design process, along with taking an evidence-based, priority informed approach. It has described some of the factors which should be considered when undertaking effective design such as leadership, resources, risk and sensitivity analysis and the issues of designing services across boundaries.

References

Boyle, D. and Harris, M. (2009) *The Challenge of Co-production: How Equal Partnerships between Professionals and the Public are Crucial to Improving Public Services*. London: NESTA.

Bubb, S. (2012) 'Opening up public services to the third sector', in N. Seddon (ed.), *The Next Ten Years*. London: REFORM.

Communities and Local Government (2011) *Best Value Statutory Guidance*. London: DCLG,

Cook, A. and Miller, E. (2012) *Talking Points – Personal Outcomes Approach: Practical Guide*. Edinburgh: Joint Improvement Team.

Department of Health (2008a) *Commissioning for Personalisation: A Framework for Local Authority Commissioners*. London: HMSO.

Department of Health Local Authority Circular (2008b) *Transforming Social Care*. London: HMSO.

DTI (2005) *Factsheet Total Quality Management (TQM)* and also http://webarchive.national-archives.gov.uk/+/www.dti.gov.uk/quality/6i.htm. Accessed 25 July 2012.

Glendinning, C., Clarke, S., Hare, P., Kotchetkova, I., Maddison, J. and Newbronner, L. (2006) *Outcomes-focused Services for Older People*. York University: Social Care Institute for Excellence.

HM Treasury (2003) *The Green Book: Appraisal and Evaluation in Central Government*. London: TSO.

HM Treasury (2006) *Varney Review: Service Transformation: A Better Service for Citizens and Business, A Better Deal for Taxpayers*. London: HMSO.

HM Treasury/Communities and Local Government (2010) *Total Place: A Whole Area Approach to Public Services*. London: HMSO.

IDeA (2006) *PMMI Project Review of Performance Improvement Models and Tools*. London: IDeA.

Lipsky, M. (1980) *Street-level Bureaucracy: Dilemmas of the Individual in Public Services*. New York: Russell Sage Foundation.

London Economics (2007) *Cost Benefit Analysis of Interventions with Parents*, DCSF Research Report DCSF-RW008. London: HMSO.

National Audit Office (2011) *Option Appraisal – Making Informed Decisions in Government*. London: NAO.

Netten, A., Beadle-Brown, J., Caiels, J., Forder, J., Malley, J., Smith, N., Trukeschitz, B., Towers, A., Welch, E. and Windle, K. (2011) *ASCOT Adult Social Care Outcomes Toolkit – Main Guidance*, V2.1, PSSRU Discussion Paper 2716/3, September. University of Kent, Canterbury: Personal Social Services Research Unit.

Radnor, Z., Walley, P., Stephens, A. and Bucci, G. (2006) *Evaluation of the Lean Approach to Business Management and its Use in the Public Sector*. Edinburgh: Scottish Executive Social Research.

RICS (2009) *Local Authority Asset Management Best Practice: Making the Right Choices*. London.

Section 3

Secure Services

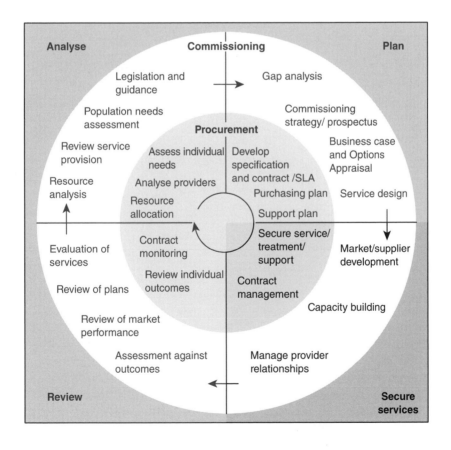

8

Market Facilitation

In 2011 Britain's care sector faced probably the biggest crisis of its history as Southern Cross, the largest provider of care homes in the UK faced bankruptcy and closure. The future funding of the care sector hit the headlines as the country faced the prospect of nearly 30,000 older people in some 750 care homes not having any security over their future care.

In the end after protracted negotiations between the Association of Directors of Adult Social Services, the owners of the care homes, the provider (Southern Cross), other providers in the care sector and government representatives, a settlement was reached. Ownership of the homes was transferred to a mixture of existing and new providers, financial arrangements were made to secure at least the short, if not the long, term future and the social care market returned once more to slumber in the national consciousness.

Yet the arrangements made over Southern Cross represented a significant milestone in the art of market facilitation of the care market. A settlement had been negotiated and agreed in which local government played a significant part, although they were neither the cause of the problems nor the provider or the direct recipients of care that was being purchased.

Learning outcomes

By the end of this chapter you should be able to:

- Understand how the public care market has developed.
- Understand the concept of market facilitation.
- Understand a three stage model around which market facilitation can be based.

Key terms

- *Block contract* – an arrangement whereby strategic commissioners pre-book a volume of care.
- *Spot contract* – purchasing care as and when required as compared to a block contract.
- *Strategic commissioning* – the act of long term planning of service provision by those responsible for an oversight of the care market.
- *Market position statement* – a concise readable document that lays out for a given market the current and future relationship between demand and supply in the market and the strategic direction that service provision might take in the future.
- *Joint strategic needs assessment* – a statutory document required to be produced by public health and the local authority that lays out the basis for need and demand for a given area.

A brief history of how the social care market has evolved

Prior to the 1980s social care in England was predominantly delivered and funded by local government. That is until the Griffiths Report, published in 1988 and enacted in the Community Care Act 1990, laid the foundations of a market in adult community care.

Parallel to the changes in adult care a similar, albeit slower change, also occurred in the externalisation of children's services particularly in the residential care sector but also in community-based provision. This has been most marked with the development of private fostering agencies and both private and voluntary sector provision for learning disability.

More controversial, but perhaps no less extensive, has been the cross party marketisation of health provision. Initially this came through the separation of purchasing or fund-holding from provision and the creation of health trusts. Increasingly the expectation now is that with the concept of health contracts going to 'any willing provider' and the purchasing decision being located with GPs more private health care providers will enter this sector.

Nonetheless it is adult social care that has led in the development of public care markets and which now plans a further shift. In 2008 the government published the circular *Transforming Social Care* (DH, 2008a) and from this, as Figure 8.1 identifies, the market embarked on another significant change.

In the future, all individuals eligible for publicly-funded adult social care will have a personal budget (other than in circumstances where people require emergency access to provision); a clear, upfront allocation of funding to enable them to make informed choices about how best to meet their needs, including their broader health and well-being.(DH, 2008a)

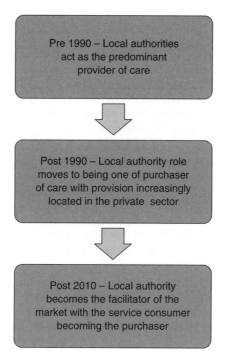

Figure 8.1   The growth of the adult social care market

Later statements such as *Commissioning for Personalisation: A Framework for Local Authority Commissioners* (DH, 2008b) began to further define the role of the local authority from one of being the dominant purchaser to a more withdrawn role:

> Traditionally councils have purchased services on behalf of their communities, tendering out contracts for providers to bid to deliver services or spot purchasing services already available in the local market. The transformation of social care demands that councils ensure the supply of the types of services and support that people need and want to buy, without the same degree of comfort from contractual arrangements. (DH, 2008b)

So what is market facilitation?

Market facilitation can be broadly defined as follows:

> Based on a good understanding of need and demand, market facilitation is the process by which strategic commissioners ensure there is sufficient appropriate provision available at the right price to meet needs and deliver effective outcomes both now and in the future.

Within the above definition a number of phrases are crucial in the interpretation of the market facilitation role as can be seen in Table 8.1.

Table 8.1 Understanding the market facilitation role

Definitional task	Application
Understanding of need and demand	In England, Health and Wellbeing boards will already have access to Joint Strategic Needs Assessments. They may also have a number of other documents that can be pulled together to give a view of demand. More advanced public care bodies will have good quality consumer research.
	However, the task is more than a simple matching of demographics to existing populations. Understanding demand is also about understanding what approaches work best, with whom and when. Where might interventions best be targeted? What situations might deteriorate leading to poor outcomes for the individual and high, potentially avoidable, costs for public care? How does strategic commissioners' understanding of demand tie in with that of actual and potential users of public care?
Sufficient appropriate provision	In the context of government policy 'sufficient' does not mean just enough, it means sufficient to offer service users some degree of choice although what constitutes choice may of course vary widely, e.g. in a rural community there may only be a single provider of dementia services (here choice may be about choice of worker, time and type of service that is delivered rather than choice of service provider).
	Equally, 'appropriate' can have a wide range of interpretations; a predominantly older person's rehabilitation service may not be appropriate for a young physically disabled adult; a meals service that does not offer a choice of menus may not be appropriate for a person who is vegetarian and from a South Asian culture.
Right price	There are likely to be a number of interpretations of what constitutes the 'right price'. 'Right' from the perspective of the purchaser and provider alike is inevitability about balancing affordability with quality and accessibility. It is not necessarily the same as cheapest. For example, if a contract price is pitched too low then the long term effect may be to limit supply and/or drive some providers out of business. Therefore, 'right' has to mean not just lowest but a price capable of delivering sustainable services of good quality.
Deliver effective outcomes	The word 'outcomes' is increasingly entering the lexicon of public care from both central and a local government. However, there remains something of a conflict between defining outcomes that it is wished a service would achieve and paying for that service by the achievement of those outcomes.
Now and in the future	Market facilitation needs to combine both short and long term strategic approaches. Of immediate concern will be day to day issues over supply and demand. However, as most providers state, the key to a successful market is about consistency of demand and price. Investment requires predictability about how the market will behave and longevity if new ideas are to mature and develop.

The case for and against facilitation

There are those who might argue that the case, particularly in social care, for commissioners facilitating the market is increasingly redundant. After all ...

- ... in adult services more people fund their own care and therefore there is less of a role for the state in intervening between consumer and provider. This is further reinforced by the growth of direct payments and personalised care which it is intended will lead to all users being purchasers of their own care.
- ... providers already know the market well. Some may have sunk all their savings into their business, therefore they don't need the health service or the local authority to tell them what is happening or what they should do.
- ... is there not a new spirit of co-production? Surely all parties should be equally involved in facilitating a public care market.

There are elements of truth in all of the above statements and there is little doubt that across many sectors of state intervention the case for moving away from a government-led command economy has long been evident. However, is a complete laissez-faire, unrestrained, market the best way of ensuring the state and the care consumer get the best possible deal? Some points to consider are:

- Many would suggest that Southern Cross should indicate greater not less state involvement in the purchase process. Certainly, the involvement of private equity firms in the provision of care is a trend which many would wish to see monitored much more closely. Few would want to see a pure market where businesses fail leaving vulnerable people without a service.
- In a pure market the tendency is always to gravitate towards larger suppliers who can offer greater economies of scale. Whilst in some aspects of public care this may be desirable there may also be a good case to protect small local organisations who supply a different kind of service.
- The majority of care purchases are still made using state funding. The duty of care and the duty to ensure such funds are spent appropriately remains with the local authority.
- Whilst personal budgets and self-directed support in the care system may increasingly be seen as significant, many people still want public care organisations to purchase or manage the purchase process on their behalf. In addition, some people lack capacity ranging from older people with dementia through to children in need of care. Research also suggests that many people make their purchase decision in an emergency or distressed circumstance, when little information is available to them.
- Finally, to achieve the end point of high quality services may require additional public sector support if innovation is to occur, if rural services and specialist care is to be financially viable and if the gap between private funded and state funded care is not to widen.

Stop and Reflect

Market facilitation is a move away from a paternalistic approach of 'the state always knows best' and into a world where strategic commissioners work with the market to ensure the sufficiency of supply of quality care is available. This process, begun in social care, is being encouraged via personal budgets in health care and across local government in terms of the whole public sector developing a more personalised approach.

The activities of market facilitation

In order to deliver this role, strategic commissioners need to embrace a range of activities. These can be summarised as:

- *Capturing and analysing market intelligence* – The development of a shared perspective of supply and demand (including identifying gaps in provision), leading to an evidenced, published, market position statement for a given market.
- *Helping to give the market structure and shape* – Creating a world where commissioners' and providers' behaviour is visible and the outcomes they are trying to achieve agreed, or at least accepted.
- *Intervening where necessary to encourage innovation and development* – The interventions commissioners make in order to encourage and stimulate the kind of market believed to be necessary for any given community.

The three functions inevitably run in tandem, possibly even independently of each other. However, this concept of facilitating the market is not new – planning authorities have been influencing the design of urban landscapes and town centres for generations – neither is it exclusive to social care or the local authority. In 2007 the World Class Commissioning Programme for health care identified stimulating the market as one of its key requirements.

PCTs will need to have in place a range of responsive providers that they can choose from. They must understand the current and future market and provider requirements. Employing their knowledge of future priorities, needs and community aspirations, PCTs will use their investment power to influence improvement, choice and service design through new or existing providers to secure the desired outcomes and quality, effectively shaping their market and increasing local choice of provision. (NHS, 2007)

Capturing and analysing market intelligence

Developing a market position statement

As the concept of market facilitation has increasingly been understood, a range of tools and materials have been developed to help build the approach. Central to this has been the creation of the concept of a market position statement (MPS).

Public care tends to have had a rich history of producing strategic documents that, in terms of their size and content, are often in an inverse relationship to their usefulness. In this instance, hopefully, the activity of capturing market intelligence, analysing the data and turning it into a market position statement will be the starting point of a dialogue with the sector and with consumers rather than simply being an end in itself. An MPS should have four substantive characteristics:

- It should be a brief analytical document that presents a picture of demand and supply now, what that might look like in the future and how strategic commissioners will support and intervene in a local market in order to deliver this vision.
- It should support its analysis by bringing together material from a range of sources such as JSNAs, surveys, market reviews and statistics into a single document which presents the data that the market needs to know if providers are to develop effective business plans.
- It is based around the market that providers define rather than how strategic commissioning is organised, e.g. older people, learning disability, etc., and cover all potential and actual users of services not just those the state funds.
- It should be a start, not the end point, of a process of market facilitation. Therefore, the MPS is the creation of strategic commissioners but if it does not present an analysis of the market that consumers and providers find useful, then it will have failed.

Table 8.2 identifies the typical content of a local authority social care MPS.

Table 8.2 The typical content of a Local Authority Social Care MPS

Developing a Market Position Statement	
A summary of the direction the local authority and its commissioning partners wish to take and the purpose of the document	• Summarises the key care and wellbeing outcomes to be achieved and any, and which, elements of policy, legislation and regulation will have an impact on the market. • Contains a summary of the key elements of the analysis presented in the individual sections below. (This section should be written last of all and ideally be no more than one page.)

(Continued)

Table 8.2 (Continued)

Developing a Market Position Statement	
The LA's predictions of future demand, identifying key pressure points	• An analysis of the current population and anticipated projections for the coming 5–10 years for the relevant market sector and the impact any population change may have on future demand for services.
	• The analysis should cover the whole population of potential service users, including those who fund services themselves and those funded by the LA either in part or in total. Consumer perspectives should be represented here.
	• Highlights particular aspects of demand now and in the future, for example, by geography (which wards have high density) and by nature of particular problems, e.g. dementia, profound and multiple disabilities, etc. and whether this is likely to increase, remain the same or diminish. This will include the rationale on which such estimates are being made.
The LA's picture of the current state of supply covering strengths and weaknesses within the market	• A review of current spend on services and in what amount.
	• A quantitative picture of supply, looking at what services are provided, to whom, where and in what volume. Particular issues to look out for could be: does the profile of service provision match likely future demand, are services located in the areas of highest need?
	• A qualitative picture of current supply indicating those areas where services appear not to be meeting required standards or users' requirements or outcomes. These may be based on reports of complaints, of user surveys, mystery shopper exercises, etc.
Identified models of practice the LA and its partners will encourage	• A review of how the commissioning organisation sees the supply side in terms of the latest evidence about the best approaches and methodologies.
	• An analysis of whether the desired models of care are matched by current provision.
	• Suggestions as to how might the market deliver change.
	• A statement about whether commissioners will continue to provide or directly purchase any services, whether it will seek framework agreements with providers or seek only to influence CQC, service users, carers, government in particular directions.
The likely future level of resourcing	• Which areas of supply the LA sees as a high priority, where it wishes to see services develop and those areas where it would be less likely to purchase or encourage service users to purchase in the future.
	• A description of likely future public care resourcing, and how this might drive the vision from the previous section.
	• If less funding is to be made available, an analysis of the likely targets which might be de-commissioned or discouraged and how the LA will seek to achieve these changes.

Developing a Market Position Statement	
The support the LA will offer towards meeting the ideal model	• An analysis of what the authority anticipates will be the impact of more service users purchasing or negotiating their own care, and the impact this might have on the market. • Any particular offers that may be available to providers, e.g. outcome-based contracts, land availability, help with planning consent, guaranteed or underwritten take up of services, training and development, business and management support, if they develop certain types of provision.

Is writing an MPS that captures and utilises the information suggested above that difficult? Well experience suggests 'yes it is'. Below are some of the aspects of an MPS that authors have struggled with:

- **Who authors?** This is a document that emanates from public care strategic commissioners. In subsequent years and versions it may represent more of a combined view of the market but initially the MPS is about the public sector laying its cards on the table. However, there should be pre-writing consultation with providers about what information do they not have that they would value and post writing, as the next section indicates, the MPS is key to structuring the market.
- **Defining a market**. This should be relatively easy but needs to be based around the providers' definition of their market not how strategic commissioners interpret different client or patient groups or disciplines. For example, there is a need to check out whether there is a cross over for the majority of providers from one client group to another. What geographical boundaries does a 'local' care market follow?
- **A document that is market facing**. This is a document for people who provide services in a particular market, whether state, private or voluntary sector. Therefore, it should give its readers information they may not already know that would be helpful in planning their future businesses, offer a clear picture of what gaps there are in the existing care market and identify what is it consumers and potential consumers are saying about services.
- **A document that is concise and readable**. In writing the MPS it is important to be clear about the distinction between description and analysis. The former, often in a health and social care context has produced long rambling commissioning strategies, where the impression is that virtue is measured by weight. It is not uncommon to hear people say 'we included it because we collected it'. An MPS should be a concise analytical document that tells us what is really important. It cuts through waffle and analyses the data that will tell us what is important about future markets and why.
- **A sharp understanding of demand**. In understanding demand, too often a simplistic view is taken of just extrapolating population data and sometimes at a great and unanalysed length. This is not likely to help providers. There are a range of factors to be taken into account, e.g., is the current trend rising or falling, are the numbers of consumers likely to be influenced by wealth or home ownership, are there factors in our population that could promote an unusually large increase or fall?

- **Covering whole populations**. In many reports, particularly in social care, strategies often only look at known and funded populations. If considering the whole market it is important to step beyond this. For example, what is the relationship between children known to have been abused and estimates of levels of abuse? What might change the balance between these? We may know how many older people are being funded by the state in residential care but how many people are self-funding and what are the future implications for the market?
- **Mapping future service provision**. It is important to be clear about what the range of provision might look like in the future, the evidence behind why this is the best approach and how this relates to future funding. There are often snap shots of good practice, but what tends to be lacking is a scaled up working model of how such case studies might fit together into a costed, whole service.

The end of the beginning

The end product of the market intelligence activity should be an evidence-based, market-facing, position statement. Typically a single sector MPS, e.g. older people or children with a learning disability, should be no more than 15 pages (concentrating on limiting size is more likely to force an analytical approach than simply producing a document that describes but does not inform). The test should always be 'how might a provider use this information?' – if this can't be answered, then don't include it!

Therefore an MPS should clearly set out:

- The overall direction strategic commissioners wish the market to take.
- Predictions of future demand across the whole market, identifying key pressure points and the rationale behind assumptions made.
- A picture of the current state of supply covering strengths and weaknesses within the market.
- The areas where strategic commissioners would wish to see services develop and those areas where it will discourage additional service provision.
- Identified models of practice commissioners will support and at what price.
- The support commissioners can offer towards innovation and development.
- What is not known? This is a new activity for most strategic commissioners and consequently there will be elements about the market that are not known. It is better to clearly state these and how such information may be sought in future rather than trying to hide up its absence.

EXERCISE 8.1

Does your MPS answer these questions about supply?

1. What is the current distribution of services in relation to the population? What does service take up look like over time?
2. Is this a market that divides into those who fund their own care and support and if so what is the distribution between the state-funded and the person-funded service?

3. What is considered to be the threshold of quality, how good is local performance as shown through complaints, CQC inspections etc?
4. Are there services that we would currently see as over or under supplied and why?
5. Have we outlined what we would consider a good service to look like, in what volumes to match demand and why have we come to that conclusion?
6. What is considered a fair price for the service on offer and what is the relationship between price and quality? If the commissioner is not offering that price what is the consequence for the service?
7. Is this a stable market, a market that is growing or a market that is in decline and what are the consequences of any of these positions?
8. Which services are financially vulnerable, which have grown and which diminished?

Does your MPS answer these questions about demand?

1. What are the broad population trends and which sectors of that population will grow the fastest, e.g. over 85s, older people with a learning disability.
2. Are there geographical distinctions in the way populations are distributed, e.g. particular areas with greater older people populations?
3. What is the relationship between the whole population and people who currently receive a service? Is it possible to distinguish between populations that are known, those that we should know and those that are likely to remain unknown?
4. Are there changes in demand that providers are experiencing and are these quantifiable, e.g. changes in the frailty and age of people being admitted to care homes?
5. Are there market sectors that will have particular problems in meeting need, e.g. dementia, strokes, people with profound and multiple disabilities etc?
6. How might past trends over time match the future trajectory of demand?
7. What surveys of the general public and of service users have been conducted? Can these be brought together with material from inspection reports and national research into clear indications about future trends and desires?
8. What sensitivity is there to price and what relationship has been established between price and service quality? Are there sectors of the market where people would be prepared to pay more for enhanced provision?

Helping to give the market structure and shape

Defining the process

The MPS may start off as a strategic commissioner's document yet it is vital that it is viewed as a calling card to both providers and consumers. As Figure 8.2 suggests, it is worth testing both the analysis and the conclusions before publicly launching the document to a wider audience.

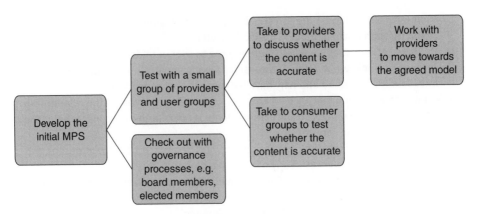

Figure 8.2 Defining the market facilitation process

As part of a wider engagement exercise a number of suggestions might be made. For example:

- Disseminate the document widely, not only to existing providers but also to organisations that have not provided in the past but might be persuaded to do so in the future.
- Be prepared to talk about the suggested strategic direction and why commissioners have come to the conclusions they have.
- Look at which forums are appropriate to discuss the document. Big events may be a good way of getting the message across to large numbers of providers in a cost effective way. However, if the desire is to have discussions about the impact the commissioning approach might have on an individual organisation it is not reasonable to expect providers to reveal their business plans and strategies to competitors.
- Is there a need to divide the discussion into smaller market segments, e.g. in the case of social care this might be home care, residential care; or into business groups such as the private sector and voluntary sector?

Potential sticking points

It is important to try and move away from price at the start of this engagement process – partly because there will be other forums for that discussion and partly because there is a need to signal that the MPS is about a different kind of relationship. Nonetheless, the relationship between price, quality and capacity is always going to be a key determinant of the size and shape of the market.

One of the common complaints from social care providers is the difference in approach the local authority adopts towards its own provision as compared to the expectations it sets for its external providers. This has become less as more services have been externalised but can still be a significant issue in some authorities. Where this occurs then the rationale for the LA remaining a provider needs to be explicit and open. There may of course be good reasons such as:

- Given geographical isolation there is no provider willing to offer a service.
- The tasks being undertaken are either so experimental and/or mission critical that the local authority or the PCT needs to provide the service.
- That commissioners wish to pilot provision before going to the market to provide a similar service.

Another frustration that providers raise is tendering in an environment where there is little indication of contract value, or where the tender processes are lengthy and resource consuming for providers but the offer at the end is only inclusion on a preferred provider list.

Where the contract is for a new type of provision and where the detail is not, or cannot be, accurately specified then commissioners run the risk of tenderers being either well wide of the mark in terms of their proposals or of providers taking on too great a risk to make their proposals sustainable. This can be reduced by better specification, by open discussions with providers and/or by a preferred provider processes.

Nonetheless, there may still be times when a LA or CCG needs to accept that it has to pay a premium to cover additional risk, where it needs to enter into partnership for provision or where it needs to provide an indication of the minimum and maximum contract value. A tendering process that does not give an indication of value does not always serve commissioners and providers well and hence may be disadvantageous in the long run to service users.

A small economic diversion

In a pure market, price acts as the fulcrum between demand and supply (demand is the amount of a good people want at a given price whilst supply is the amount of a good on offer at that price). If demand falls and supply remains constant or increases then the price falls. If demand rises and supply remains the same or diminishes then prices rise. There are those who argue this is how care markets should work independent of state intervention.

Strategic commissioners when they act as purchasers either through block or spot purchasing contracts or through limiting the amount of money available in direct payments and personal budgets, distort the purity of the market. The price they are prepared to pay is often independent of whether demand or supply is rising or falling but instead is based on the amount of funding they have at their disposal. If commissioners push prices down and costs remain high or increase, it has a significant impact on suppliers. Whilst this may be survivable in the short term particularly if it was felt that the previous price paid was too high, in the longer term it could potentially have the opposite effect:

- Prices might increase because a number of care businesses fail and hence there is a greater shortage of supply. This will drive up price and give providers greater control over the market.

(Continued)

(Continued)

- There will be increasing price demarcation between self-funders and those who are state funded. State-funded care purchasers will only get the service capacity left after self-funders have had their demands met.
- The quality of service is reduced, e.g. wages are capped and training not undertaken to reduce costs. In the case of residential care larger and larger homes are developed to warehouse people at a lower price per head.
- If the manufacturing and service sectors economically recover before the public sector this is likely to lead to a labour shortage in the public sector which will again inflate price.

Structuring activities

Assessing the impact of price

As stated above, many of the past relationships in social care, between providers and strategic commissioners, have focused around price, costs, terms and conditions. There is clearly a balance to be struck between the short term and long term approaches to managing the relationship between these factors. The best approach is to come up with an agreed structure for calculating a fair price for care. This means that providers will know what will be taken into account in calculating their costs and can plan for the future

Business planning

It is fairly obvious that commissioners need to know what providers are planning for the future so that there is a reasonable chance that the services users may wish to take up, are going to be in place. Having said that, the impression given by commissioning organisations is that few seem to have made attempts to discuss with providers their business plans or assist smaller providers in developing them. Failure to do this might mean smaller but valued providers fail because they don't plan appropriately, that opportunities for innovation are lost or of providers over extending their services in a way that is not sustainable.

Implementing personalisation

It will be vitally important to identify with providers how service users' choice can be developed and improved and to monitor the impact that direct payments and personal budgets are having on the sector. This will be equally true in health care for personal health budgets. It is important to note that personalisation of services does not automatically exclude block contracts (which may through guaranteeing provision mean consumers can have a wider choice of times, services and care workers).

Assessing viability

Provider vulnerability may arise through a range of circumstances. Over commitment in agreeing to a contract that is not financially sustainable, changes in interest rates or labour costs, changes in personnel, or too great a demand that cannot be controlled, may all be factors that can make a provider vulnerable. It is important that commissioners understand the nature of such vulnerability, do not acerbate it through harsh tendering processes and identify which organisations may need support and how it can best be offered. Where vulnerability occurs because the service is no longer desired by service users it may still be important that the resource in terms of people or premises or organisation are not lost to the social care sector. Therefore, having an early warning of the need to change the product and offering help in restructuring may be beneficial.

Providing an innovative environment

The need for support might not come about just through vulnerability but also through an organisation's potential strength. Innovation may occur because existing products are suffering lower demand, through a provider wishing to increase their market share or through changing consumer expectations. However, innovation also implies risk. Where innovation is desired, providers and strategic commissioners should work together to determine how risk can be reduced.

Encouraging diversity

Some new developments may arise through diversification by existing providers. For example, registered housing providers, recognising the increasing age of their tenants might be encouraged to explore how they can begin to offer other services that can sustain people within the community, e.g. care and repair services. A care home may diversify into offering a wider range of outreach services into the community.

Following on from developing an MPS consider whether you have:

1. Consulted on and published the market position statement?
2. Actively promoted the model of what the range of care should look like based on good practice?

(Continued)

EXERCISE 8.2

(Continued)

3. Been clear where and why the LA is a provider? Diminished differences between in-house and external systems where these potentially compete in the same market?
4. Identified with other parts of the LA or health service how well any local environment and community is configured in order to ensure that potential health and social care needs can be met?
5. Reviewed tendering and procurement processes, evaluated their impact on provider communities and explored how improvements can be made that will help drive the market?
6. Developed an awareness of providers' long term business plans and where future support might be needed? Identified business cycles across the third and private sectors?
7. Worked with providers to assess the impact that greater choice, via personal budgets and direct payments, might have on costs and availability of service provision?
8. Identified how commissioners can reduce the vulnerability of valued providers?
9. Identified where there are barriers to market entry where new resources are needed and identified with providers how these might be overcome?
10. Looked for potential diversification amongst existing organisations, e.g. can RSLs do care and repair, can home care agencies deliver assistive technology?
11. Developed a process for monitoring the impact of the MPS, reviewing the data it contains and updating?

Market intervention

This final section looks at those instances where strategic commissioners may need or want to intervene in a market in order to directly support particular activities and innovations. Such interventions may take place because strategic commissioners have identified:

- There is a gap in service provision which is unlikely to be filled unless they directly intervene.
- They need to try and avoid the possibility of local monopolistic supply.
- They want to encourage providers to offer a different type of service.
- They want to encourage a wider range of providers and recognise that entering the market may be difficult and that small organisations need help and support if they are to grow and be successful.

Active support to providers

The preceding section identified how commissioners might start to shape, structure and influence the direction that the market takes. However, such activities alone may not offer the diversity of supply and choice that is needed. Sometimes the support from commissioning bodies needs to be more active. This may be through positive initiatives such as help with business planning, grant aid or guaranteed contracts which will underwrite supply. It may also come through removing barriers to market entry, through lessening complex tendering processes, reducing planning controls, or making land and premises more widely available. Some of these factors are explored in more detail below.

Example: Intervening in the housing market

Most local authorities not only have an ageing population but also an older people's population that is wealthier through occupational pensions and housing equity (half of all housing equity is held by people aged 65 and over). Yet the widespread development of a range of housing for sale suitable for older people has hardly occurred.

Faced with any level of incapacity most older people either 'make do' in their existing family home, move to rented and often outdated sheltered housing or go into residential care. Yet there is a wealth of evidence which shows that if older people move to property suitable to needs there is a substantial health and care gain.

Strategic commissioners could intervene to stimulate, particularly the private market, through:

- Working with registered and private sector providers to review existing sheltered housing stock and develop a joint plan for redevelopment.
- Providing a programme of interest free loans in order to stimulate the market.
- Arranging for staggered repayment where LA land is used for development.
- Arranging a programme of information for local architects and developers about extra care housing which can boost the local construction economy.
- Ensuring that the planning authority fully understands future demand from older people, the financial gain that retirement housing offers and the volume in which it might be needed.

Most of these interventions are fairly small scale but may just tip the balance between having a buoyant and a stagnant market.

Business support

Many local authorities have had or still have business support initiatives and are actively involved in regeneration of one sort or another. Yet somehow social care and health care often gets left behind in these initiatives despite the economic contribution social care makes to localities and in many areas is one the biggest employers. It may be particularly valuable where people seek part time work or wish to work irregular hours. Therefore a wider discussion about the future role of the public care sector and the part it plays in the local economy across all council functions could well be a helpful prelude to any interventions.

Planning

Of particular importance where the delivery of care involves buildings, will be the local planning system. Discussion here may centre on the balance of different types of provision. Given the intended localisation of planning is there a need for supplementary guidance in order to discourage providers in sectors where there is already an oversupply of certain types of provision?

In the past most commissioners have tended to see planning interventions simply in terms of Section 106 agreements of the Town and Country Planning Act (1990) where either the local authority is seeking to gain some additional social investment through granting planning permission or to constrain developers from making changes to a building or environment that might be considered detrimental. However, to a new or small social care business, the planning system can act as a major deterrent to investment and help in navigating planning processes from the local authority may be most welcome. It certainly suggests that at the very least the market structure plan should be discussed with planning colleagues.

Training

Clearly where commissioners want providers to adopt a particular approach or change the basis of its contracts with either the commissioning body or with individuals then there is a need to train staff and managers to ensure that this can be successfully achieved. This may be particularly true where the desire is to change the focus of intervention and the measures of performance from outputs onto outcomes. Such an approach requires much greater expertise in understanding the relationship between issues or problems and intervention and much greater flexibility in working practice. For example, in the case of home care staff it may require employing people with not only a wider range of skills and at higher cost but also with a greater ability to recognise key conditions that may affect older people.

Brokerage

Following on from exploring vulnerability as part of the market intelligence activities, there may be actions that commissioners would wish to take in order to safeguard key services. For example if two organisations perform similar functions but both are too small to remain viable it may be helpful to broker discussions between them in order to develop shared working. If vulnerability arises from the provider having agreed contract terms that make the business unviable there may be a need to renegotiate those conditions. Obviously, commissioners need to approach the market in an even handed way and not be seen to give preferential benefits to one supplier over another; on the other hand if a diverse market offering good quality services and choice to service users is to be created then different types of support are likely to be needed by individual providers. Even handedness should never be used as a reason why a needed and irreplaceable service could not survive.

Active intervention for consumers

Market intervention may also of course occur in terms of interventions that directly support consumers of services to strike a better arrangement with providers and to push expectations of public care. In the past PCTs and the local authority have tended to rely on complaints or questionnaires in order to obtain the views of service users. There are a number of problems with this approach:

- Complaints and surveys tend to be passive, they rely on the user expressing a view rather than actively seeking to know how the service could be better and encouraging open criticism.
- People tend to be constrained by what they feel is possible or by what they know is available. It is hard to be creative in thinking of a new approach that does not exist, particularly in a climate where health and social care staff may regularly be telling service users how hard pressed they are and services are often distressed purchases.
- Many processes for testing the views of users tend to be confined to people who receive state support rather than surveys that cover self-funders, so the overall picture tends to be biased and partial.
- Many people find it hard to complain when they may be dependent on that agency or individual for the delivery of a service that is highly personal, e.g. washing, bathing or helping people to the toilet.

Therefore, a key part of market facilitation should be about the local authority or Clinical Commissioning Group delivering market research about current and future trends in demand. Intervention in this way helps to create a pool of unbiased knowledge which both current and potential providers might use in order to make their decisions about future provision. It is also important in giving consumers an accurate view about services as well as informing strategic commissioners about how they should influence the market in future.

However, market intervention for consumers can take a number of other forms.

- Giving help to people to make their own purchase decisions through direct payments, through registers of personal assistants (PAs), through stimulating the PA role as a job opportunity and providing training to PAs.
- Making information better available. Increasingly people are getting used to the idea, via the internet, that before making a major purchase decision it is possible to see what other people have made of the product, whether that is buying a new car or holiday or computer. The care sector is one of the few areas where making a major purchase decision does not

have this kind of consumer facility. Local authorities may wish to commission a third party to create consumer websites.

- At the time of writing some local authorities are exploring their own care insurance schemes as is at least one extra care housing provider.
- At the time of writing one local authority is working with independent financial advisors to ensure that self-funders of residential care are getting good quality information about their savings and investments.

Potential market intervention activities

1. Refocus local authority business support initiatives onto the health and social care market.
2. Explore how local projects can attract capital investment and what guarantees may be needed.
3. Develop social enterprise organisations.
4. Explore where planning barriers exist and negotiate how that process can be improved for providers.
5. Offer access to training that commissioners and providers agree can improve performance.
6. Promote local 'Which type?' care guides which emphasise a consumer perspective.
7. Help to broker consolidation of the market where there are gains to be made from small businesses becoming less vulnerable.
8. Offer purchase documentation for individual service users/carers to use.
9. Ensure standard frameworks and contracts are used that are fair to purchasers and providers.

Summary

The age of the public care market being dominated by monopolistic purchasers of care is gradually coming to an end through the growth of self-funders and increased devolution of state funding to consumers. At the same time the role of strategic commissioners in ensuring sufficiency of good quality care services becomes even more crucial. This calls for diversity.

At times it will be right to purchase services via an overall block contract, to recognise that individual purchasers need good quality information but sometimes want someone else to take those decisions for them. Equally, strategic commissioners may need to recognise and carry the battle within their own organisations that focusing on short term price may in the end cost the public sector more. Choice needs to be defined by the consumer not by commissioners who may only see choice in terms of a choice of provider.

Above all else the transformation of public care will only take place with and through the market. Those commissioners who choose to see themselves as all powerful purchasers may be in for a rude awakening in the coming years.

References

Department of Health (2008a) *Transforming Social Care*. London: HMSO.
Department of Health (2008b) *Commissioning for Personalisation: A Framework for Local Authority Commissioners*. London: HMSO.
NHS (2007) *World Class Commissioning Programme*. London: HMSO.

9
Procurement and the Contracting Process

Commissioners have many tools at their disposal to achieve the best outcomes possible for the resources available. This often involves the use of procurement to obtain new services or to change existing provider arrangements. With more and more public services opened up to a wider range of providers (HM Government, 2012b), the need for commissioners to understand procurement and the contracting process is ever more important.

This chapter explores the key elements of procurement and contracting and how these approaches can be used throughout the commissioning cycle to ensure that value for money is obtained and that outcomes for users of services are delivered efficiently and effectively.

Learning outcomes

By the end of this chapter you should be able to:

- Describe what procurement and contracting are.
- Summarise the main legislation and regulations surrounding procurement and contracting.
- Identify opportunities for strategic procurement to improve value for money.
- Describe the key steps of the contracting process.

Key terms

- *Contract* – a binding agreement made between two or more parties, which is intended to be enforceable in law.

> • *Procurement* – the process of acquiring goods, works or services from, usually, exter-
> nal providers and managing these through to the end of contract. It also includes
> the strategic activities that support this process.

What is procurement and when is it used?

Procurement is the process of acquiring goods, works or services from, usually, external providers and suppliers and managing these through to the end of contract. For ease of reference, in this chapter the term 'services' will be used to describe 'goods, works or services' and 'providers' will be used to describe both 'providers and suppliers'.

Procurement can involve both strategic procurement activities such as an analysis of expenditure or 'spend analysis' across the organisation, and the management of the contracting process for specific services including specification writing, inviting tenders and managing a contract.

The relationship between commissioning and procurement is set out in the IPC commissioning model described in Chapter 1. Alternatively the commissioner may use grants, joint funding with a partner organisation or personalised service provision such as direct payments. Contracting for personalised services is considered in detail in Chapter 10.

Nevertheless, the importance placed on procurement in the public sector has grown over the years as services have increasingly been outsourced with the intention to secure value for money. All local authorities and a range of other organisations in the public sector are under a general duty of best value to 'make arrangements to secure continuous improvement in the way in which its functions are exercised, having regard to a combination of economy, efficiency and effectiveness' (Department for Communities and Local Government, 2011a: 6).

A potential advantage of procurement is that it can introduce competition, so that commissioners have a range of service providers to choose from. This can help them to make more informed decisions about services that provide value for money as well as encouraging providers to ensure their offers are a good buy (Department for Education, n.d. a).

The notion of competition in the public sector has been further advanced by the desire to open up public services (HM Government 2011, 2012a). One key aspect of this policy initiative is to widen the number of providers of public services and to reduce the amount of services run internally. For example, some local authorities are increasingly seeing themselves as 'commissioning organisations' rather than providers of services. Newton (2011) aptly summarises the thinking that underpins this agenda:

Open Public Services is based on the theory that market competition between providers improves the quality of services experienced by service users, and will make them more effective, thereby improving social outcomes, and reducing costs. It identifies an important new role for government as that of having responsibility for ensuring free competition.

Although the current policy drive is to open up public services, commissioners need to consider the advantages and disadvantages of procuring services. For most businesses there is a 'make or buy' decision to be made (e-notes, 2012). Reasons procurement may not be suitable could include the need for very close control and management of the services provided, risks associated with having to change providers at the end of the contract period and the cost of procurement compared to the potential gains. The cost of procurement can be significant for both providers and the purchasing organisation; for example, Dudkin and Välilä (2005) found that, for a sample of 25 hospital PFI procurements in the UK, the transaction costs for the public sector and the winning bidder were some 8% of the total capital investment cost. Commissioners need to be aware that providers may seek to recoup the costs associated with the procurement and that this is likely to affect how proposals are costed.

Another reason for not considering procurement may be the lack of providers in the market place, and market activities (see Chapter 8) may be required before embarking on procurement, to ensure sufficient capability, capacity and competition.

There will however be many reasons why procurement may be seen as advantageous (e-notes, 2012). Examples include:

- A lack of in-house expertise.
- Services are cheaper to buy than to produce.
- More service choice is needed.
- Insufficient capacity in-house.
- Cheaper to buy services when they are needed rather than have fixed cost.
- Specialist small volume services are required.
- Encourages innovation in service provision.

Stop and Reflect

Think about the advantages and disadvantages of procuring services in your service area.

As a commissioner you may have to fundamentally rethink how you deliver services because of changes in needs and available resources. Might procurement be able to help you with this?

If commissioning leads to a decision to procure services, it is important that commissioners are aware of the procurement rules that apply to public bodies. For example, if a commissioner is working closely with providers throughout the commissioning cycle, it is essential to be clear about when a formal procurement process has begun so that the procurement is lawful, fair and transparent (Cook et al., 2009).

Procurement can be complex and it is a heavily regulated area of work, so it is advisable that commissioners involve procurement expertise as early as possible in the commissioning process and in procurement activities. Although the commissioner will ensure that the whole commissioning exercise is project managed from beginning to end, getting solid procurement advice will help to ensure compliance with rules and regulations and that maximum benefit is obtained from any procurement.

Legislation, regulatory framework and guidance

There is a range of legislation and guidance that governs procurement in any public organisation.

EU procurement directives

Firstly, procurement has to be compliant with the European Union (EU) Procurement regulations that apply across the whole of the European Union. Where the regulations apply, failure to comply with these rules may lead to challenge through the courts. Procurement rules consist of:

- EU Treaty – the EU public procurement market is a fundamental part of the single market and is governed by rules intended to remove barriers and open up new, non-discriminatory and competitive markets for companies.
- EU procurement directives – establish detailed rules governing the award of public contracts over set thresholds.
- EU remedies directives – require that member states provide rapid and effective remedies for breach of the rules.

Service contracts are divided into two categories:

- Part A – to which the full EU rules apply.
- Part B – where the only obligations relate to non-discriminatory technical specifications, and notice of contract award. There is no requirement for contracts to be advertised in the *Official Journal of the EU* (OJEU), but Part B services should be subject to some form of appropriate advertised competition.

Health and social services are Part B services; however, it is worth noting that this categorisation relates to what is being bought rather than who is doing the buying. For example an Adult Social Care department advertising a contract for a transport service would be considered a Part A service and the full EU rules would apply (National Market Development Forum, 2011). Look out for

European Commission proposals to change the procurement directives including which services fall into 'Part B', expected to come into force in June 2014.

The regulations only apply if the contract is over a threshold amount and differs for supplies, services and works and whether the purchasing body is central government or another public sector organisation. The threshold is updated every 2 years.

There are EU rules for the valuation of contracts and care is therefore required. The contract value to be employed for the purposes of the thresholds is the estimated contract value, not annual value, and contracting authorities are required to aggregate the value of related or connected contracts. In any event, contracting authorities are prohibited from 'splitting' contracts with the intention of avoiding the directives.

Under the EU procurement rules there is a choice of four procurement award procedures (Office for Government Commerce, 2008) that can be used:

- *Open procedure.* This is a one-stage process where the invitation to tender is advertised and all interested providers can submit their bids. All bids are then evaluated.
- *Restricted procedure.* This is the most commonly used procedure (Cook et al., 2009). It is a two-stage process where a short list is drawn up from those that have responded to an advert, usually by using a pre-qualification questionnaire (PQQ). The types of questions that may be used in PQQs are limited by the procurement directives but generally focus on the providers' legal and financial status and their management and technical capability to deliver the required service. In order to reduce the burden in particular on small providers, there is a drive to standardise PQQs and many organisations, such as central government departments use preset questions. Once the short list is finalised, selected providers are invited to tender. This procedure avoids having to evaluate an overwhelmingly large number of tenders.
- *Competitive dialogue procedure.* This procedure can only be used in strictly defined, exceptional circumstances where purchasers consider that the open or restricted procedures will not allow the award of the contract. It is intended for use in particularly complex contracts where purchasers may be aware of needs but do not know in advance what is the best technical, legal or financial solution for satisfying them.
- *Negotiated procedure.* There are strict rules about negotiation with prospective providers under the other procedures but this procedure specifically allows negotiation with a single or a few select bidders The negotiated procedure can be used when the nature or risk involved are such that it does not permit prior overall pricing, or a specification cannot be drawn up with precision to allow the open or restricted procedure. In certain circumstances the contract does not have to be advertised under the negotiated procedure, unlike the others.

Where the value of services to be procured falls below the EU threshold value, or is a Part B service, there is still a requirement to ensure that procurement is transparent, and that potential suppliers are treated equally and in non-discriminatory way.

National legislation and guidance

The second area governing procurement is national legislation and statutory guidance. The Public Contracts Regulations 2006, the Public Contract (Amendment) Regulations 2009 and the Public Procurement (Miscellaneous Amendments) Regulations 2011 give effect in UK law to the EU procurement directives. The first two regulations do not apply to Scotland, where similar regulations exist. Case law is continuously evolving as a result of the judgements of the European Court of Justice and national UK courts which interpret EU and national law.

In recent years a significant emphasis has been placed on increasing the transparency of how public money is being spent. Local authorities are expected to publish data online of all public spend over £500, and each year authorities have to open up their accounting records for public inspection within 20 working days. As set out in *The Code of Recommended Practice for Local Authorities on Data Transparency* (Department for Communities and Local Government, 2011b), authorities are expected to publish copies of contracts and tenders to businesses and voluntary community and social enterprise organisations, as well as to itemise clearly and list grants to the latter.

The *Statutory Best Value Guidance* (Department for Communities and Local Government, 2011a) sets out the duty of best value and stipulates what authorities should do when considering reducing or ceasing funding to voluntary organisations and small businesses. There is a requirement to give at least three months notice of the reduction to be made to the organisation concerned, as well as informing service users and the public. Authorities should also involve the provider and service users before the decisions are made and allow them to put forward alternative options.

The guidance also states the need to consider value in the broadest sense including economic, environmental and social value, when service provision is reviewed.

The Public Service (Social Value) Act 2012 sets out how public authorities are required to have regard to economic, social and environmental wellbeing in connection with public services contracts and in related procurement activities. This legislation states that authorities must consider:

- How what they are proposing to procure might improve the economic, social and environmental wellbeing of the relevant area.
- How in the process of the procurement it might act with a view to secure that improvement.

However, the authority must consider only matters that are relevant to what is proposed to be procured and, in doing so, must consider the extent to which it is proportionate in all the circumstances to take those matters into account.

The Equality Act 2010, which established a new general equality duty, also applies to procurement by public authorities and is extended to providers that are contracted, and this enables authorities to use procurement to push equality objectives (Bevan Brittan, 2012; IdeA, 2012).

Internal processes and policies

Finally, all local authorities and NHS organisations have their own standing orders and scheme of financial delegation. Commissioners need to familiarise themselves with these documents. For instance, a local authority will have their own set rules about how many quotes are required for a certain amount of spend and when requirements should be put out for tender. The organisation's financial scheme of delegation will set out who in the organisation can make decisions about spend. This will often vary according to the sums of money involved: for example, large contracts may need approval from a Director or Elected Members, whereas a small spot purchase may be undertaken by a junior officer.

Many organisations also have written guidance on how procurement should be undertaken and commissioners will need to refer to these when engaging in procurement activities.

Stop and Reflect

- Find out what written guidance your organisation has on procurement policy and procedures.
- Review if internal rules are outdated or restrict the ability to procure effectively and efficiently. If change is needed, what can you do to improve internal processes and policies?

Strategic procurement

Increasingly, organisations in the public sector are taking a strategic approach to manage procurement in order to streamline procurement processes and to ensure that value for money is maximised. There may be a central or departmental team in the organisation that specialises in procurement and it is vital for commissioners to build strong links with their procurement colleagues so that opportunities for strategic procurement are identified and that procurement initiatives support commissioning.

If there is a significant increase in the amount of procurement undertaken, it may be advisable to review the organisational structure to ensure that sufficient skills and capacity are available to both procure services and to manage subsequent contracts.

Any shift in the approach to procurement, such as a reduction in grant giving in favour of procurement, can impact substantially on providers who may not be geared up to new procedures. To alleviate some of these potential difficulties some public sector bodies work with businesses and the voluntary and community sector, to ensure that providers are able to bid for business, for example, by supporting infrastructure organisations or by providing written advice and information events.

A central aspect of strategic procurement is to have an overarching approach across the organisation with clear governance arrangements and documents that set out plans and processes. Many organisations publish commissioning and procurement strategies and plans to support their strategic approach to procurement. Some local authorities have also started to provide market position statements aimed at providers to stimulate an effective market (see Chapter 8).

In order to avoid omitting crucial core conditions when contracting for services, many organisations have developed standard terms and conditions of contract. These should be included in invitations to tender and it is advisable not to sign up to a provider's terms and conditions if this can be avoided.

There are a range of strategic procurement tools that commissioners and procurement staff can use and some of the main ones are described below.

A fundamental step for many strategic procurement activities is to undertake a *spend analysis*. This involves gathering detailed data regarding how money is spent in the organisation. Examples of issues to be reviewed during the analysis include:

- What is being bought?
- How much is spent with different providers?
- Who is spending the money?
- Are there variations in unit costs?
- What are the most expensive services?

This information can then be used to identify opportunities for targeted procurement activities to increase value for money. It may for example identify areas where there are several contracts with one provider at different prices, or where too many different providers are being used.

Spend analysis is an important step in *category management*. Category management involves a process of categorising services and then managing these categories as 'business units'. For example, a category could be 'residential placements for looked after children'. Category management is normally focused on high spend/high risk categories and commissioners, procurers and other stakeholders work together to fully understand their requirements and the market, and to develop a strategy for driving value for money. Category management has been adopted by several councils and many of the techniques used will be familiar to commissioners.

Strategies developed as part of the category management may identify areas where *collaborative procurement* could be advantageous. Collaborative procurement is when organisations or departments get together to procure services. By aggregating spend it may be possible to have greater influence over quality and price. For example, district councils in Warwickshire and Worcestershire under-took a spend analysis, which helped them identify several areas for collaborative procurement, such as agency staff (Haslam, n.d.).

Framework agreements are a useful tool to support collaborative procurement as they provide opportunities to achieve economies of scale. These are pre-tendered agreements and can be set up with one or several providers. Requirements are 'called-off' as required thereby reducing the procurement effort. The agreement is for a specific time period and the provider has to deliver goods and services when requested.

More advanced procurement organisations are adopting *e-procurement tools*. These can help to reduce costs and speed up processes. Tools include web por-tals for advertising and submitting tenders, e-market places for ordering and processing invoices, and contract management packages. Some authorities have used e-auctions to procure goods and services, for example, in the West Midlands, several local authorities have used the approach to procure school transport (Improvement and Efficiency West Midlands, n.d.).

Stop and Reflect

- Jot down examples of strategic procurement in your own organisation and consider whether there may be opportunities to undertake other strategic procurement activities.

CASE STUDY

A local authority was experiencing a significant increase in their spend on fostering and residential placements for looked after children (LAC). The primary cause of this was two fold: firstly an increase in the number of LAC; and secondly an increasing shortage of in-house fostering placements, which the local authority in the past had been able to provide at a lower cost than externally bought placements. The budget pressure was also of great concern as consideration had to be given to redirecting money from early intervention and prevention work to fund the overspend. However, the authority was very reluctant to take this course of action as potentially over time this would only serve to increase the number of looked after children. It was also com-mitted to ensuring that children and young people should as far as possible be placed in their local area.

To deal with the overspend, the authority set up a working group that developed a LAC action plan. This plan contained a wide variety of actions ranging from activities to prevent children becoming looked after, increased support for LA foster carers to stem the declining numbers of in-house placements, and plans to procure agency LAC place-ments differently. Traditionally, all placements had been bought on a spot purchased basis when no suitable in-house placement could be found.

Firstly the authority took a category management approach to the procurement of residential placements. Following a very detailed analysis of the market, a decision was made to invite tenders for a 5 year contract for a 4 bed residential unit for young people aged 15–18. The contract was awarded to an existing local provider and cost savings of 20% per placement were achieved compared to the cost of spot purchasing individual placements. Overall, the new arrangement has worked well, as it has reduced the number of young people who have to move out of the area when in need of a placement. The arrangement has given the provider more financial stability which has translated into the reduced cost per placement.

Secondly, the authority decided to join forces with a neighbouring authority and set up a 3 year framework agreement for fostering placements. The framework is for placements for children with disabilities, sibling groups and for children and young people over the age of 10. Again, savings have been achieved as the unit cost is lower and also the transaction costs in finding suitable placements have been reduced.

Lessons learnt include the need to have a thorough needs assessment to direct the commissioning and procurement activities so that it is very clear what services need to be bought and providers are very clear about the services required. Secondly, the need to forecast demand, both to estimate the value size of the framework agreement and to award a long term contract with fixed costs. Finally, when working in partnership with another authority it is important to invest time in establishing good working relationships to ensure good cooperation throughout the lifetime of the framework agreement, and to ensure that the benefits of the agreement are available to both authorities.

Question

What were the strategic procurement activities that the local authority undertook, and what other actions could they have undertaken?

The contracting process

A commissioning process may result in a decision to buy services. For low value purchasing, most organisations have simplified rules, but for higher spend a more formal and regulated approach is required to comply with rules and regulations and to ensure that any procurement is fair and transparent. This is often referred to as the contracting process.

The 10-stage approach to the contracting process set out in Figure 9.1 has been developed by the Department for Education (n.d. b). The model outlines very much the same approach shown earlier in the inner circle of the commissioning cycle, although that figure is presented differently and provides a more detailed stepped approach to the contracting task. The model highlights the importance of managing the contract process as a project and shows how learning from contracted services needs to feed into future commissioning decisions.

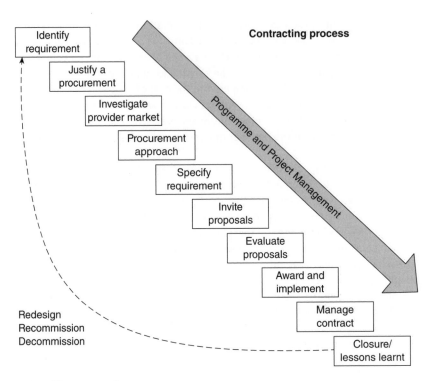

Figure 9.1   The contracting process

Source: Department of Education

www.gov.uk/government/organisations/department-for-education/about/procurement

Some of the main tasks for each step are described below to provide a brief introduction to the contracting process. Commissioners who are planning to undertake procurement are advised to seek out more detailed guidance (see section at the end of this chapter for further reading and web resources) and to ensure that they are supported by procurement experts in their organisation throughout the process.

Identify a requirement

Following the 'analyse' and 'planning' stage of the commissioning process, commissioners should be able to specify what the commissioning intentions are and what outcomes are being sought.

At this point it may also be useful to consider wider social, economic and environmental factors that need to be taken into account.

Justify a procurement

Having identified a requirement, commissioners need to consider different options to achieve the required services. An options appraisal (see Chapter 5) can help to fully evaluate if procurement is the right way forward. If a decision is made to go down the procurement route, think about the timescales required and identify who needs to be involved at the different stages of the process. For more complex procurements develop a fully costed business case and set up a project team with clear roles and responsibilities. As well as commissioners, procurement and service representatives also consider including others such as HR, pensions and property experts.

Investigate the provider market

The work involved at this stage will vary according to what needs to be bought and the existing knowledge of the relevant market.

In particular it will be useful to gather information about the capacity of the market and number of potential providers, relevant price information and potential interest from providers to bid for the contract. Actions to stimulate the market may be required and detailed information regarding market facilitation can be found in Chapter 8 of this book.

Define the procurement approach

The first step is to establish the potential value of the procurement and which rules and regulations apply. Explore opportunities for collaboration, and find out if existing framework agreements held internally or by other organisations could be utilised. There is a range of professional buying organisations in the public sector and it is worth investigating if they have framework agreements that can be used.

Also make a judgement about whether one provider or several are needed, and consider the potential advantages and disadvantages of breaking up a contract into smaller lots to encourage smaller providers to bid, or to encourage consortia bids and allowing sub contracting.

Think carefully about what is most likely to secure value for money. If the EU rules apply, find out which procurement award procedures can be used and decide which one is most suitable. Also, address issues such as: What should the length of contract be? How should performance be awarded? Would it be useful to be open with providers about the budget available?

Specify the requirement

Develop a written specification which sets out what is required so that potential providers are able to provide a costed proposal. The specification will form part of the contract so great care needs to be taken. Cover areas such as: outcomes to be achieved; required outputs and non negotiable expectations; monitoring of performance; payments and whether there are any performance related incentives; and expectations of the provider when the contract comes to an end. Also ensure that business continuity and exit requirements are included.

Once the specification has been finalised, draft the evaluation criteria that will be used to evaluate the proposals. Decide the weightings of the different criteria in order to enable a decision to be made on which proposal offers best value for money. Work with stakeholders to develop the specification and evaluation criteria to ensure both documents reflect the outcomes being sought.

There is a growing interest in outcome-focused specifications, and one advantage is that they can encourage providers to innovate. In addition, payments by results are being introduced in a range of service areas as a way to incentivise providers to deliver desired outcomes.

Take time to develop a Pricing Schedule, i.e. a template which tenderers fill in to show how they are going to charge you. This can be used to shape providers' thinking about charges.

Invite proposals

The invitation to tender documents need to include, for example, the specification, the evaluation criteria, pricing schedule and standard contract terms and conditions (in relation to the value and type of contract). In particular ensure that aspects such as intellectual property rights, termination of contract and TUPE arrangements are covered, and that there are no discrepancies between the specification and the terms and conditions.

Advertise if necessary with good notice via a sufficiently accessible advert, e.g. the organisation's website, regional portal websites, Supply2.gov.uk or OJEU. Take care to ensure that any advertisement truly reflects the specification and provide contact details for any queries. Sometimes organisations organise information events regarding specific tenders where potential providers can ask questions. Ensure that information provided in response to any queries is available to all potential providers to ensure a fair and transparent process. Where possible, send invitations to tender to a range of suitable providers.

Shortlist if necessary. If the restricted procedure is used, this step is a two-stage process where a shortlist of providers is drawn up following the use of pre-qualifying questionnaires. If appropriate, short listing can also be used for part B services or for procurement under the threshold value.

Evaluate proposals

Once the closing date has passed, evaluate tenders against the pre-agreed evaluation criteria. If possible involve a selection of stakeholders in the evaluation process, including users of the service. If needed, interview potential providers to seek clarification on the proposal that they have submitted, but make sure that no new additional evaluation criteria are introduced. The award of the contract should be on the basis of 'most economically advantageous' to the purchaser rather than lowest price.

Award and implement the contract

Before awarding the contract make sure the budget is available and that there is clarity about what is being signed up to in the contract. The award should be in writing and ensure that it is clearly recorded which documents form part of the contract. If the procurement falls within the EU directives send the *Post Award Notification*. Provide unsuccessful tenderers with feedback.

Manage the contract

Contracts need to be managed, and performance should be regularly reviewed and monitored as set out in the contract. The basis of this should be set out in the contract and included in the tenderers' costs. Chapter 11 of this book provides detailed information on performance management.

If possible develop good working relationships with the providers and encourage innovation and service improvements. Risks should be managed and it is sensible to have contingency plans in place in case problems develop with the contract.

Ask providers to contribute to needs assessments, and start planning for future commissioning or decommissioning well ahead of the end of the contract. Develop exit strategies, and don't forget to give notices for the end of contract if required.

Closure/lessons learnt

Make sure the learning from each procurement exercise is captured to ensure ongoing improvement in the organisation's procurement practice and influence future strategic procurement activities.

Stop and Reflect

- What are the strengths and weaknesses of the contract process in your own organisation?

Tips for successful procurement and contracting

To ensure that any procurement exercise reaps maximum benefits and that decisions made can stand up to any potential scrutiny, the following tips may be of assistance:

- Be clear about what needs to be purchased and what outcomes are being sought. Make sure this accords with the commissioning strategy for the service area or user group.
- Use project management tools to manage the procurement exercise; this will help to ensure for example that any statutory time requirements are adhered to and that risks are identified early on.
- Involve procurement specialists as early as possible in the process to make sure the procurement is compliant with rules and regulations and that the procurement process is used to best effect to maximise the desired outcomes.
- Clarify who will manage the contract for the service at the outset and involve them in the procurement process. For example, ask for their advice in specifying how the contract will be monitored.
- Draw on the expertise of all stakeholders and involve them where possible in the process. For example, involve service users in drawing up service specifications, evaluating tenders and monitoring of contracts.
- Innovate – use outcomes-based specifications if possible, pick evaluation criteria that support the desired outcomes, build trusting relationships with providers and consider the use of incentives, e.g. payment by results.
- Understand the market and speak to providers, but make sure unfair advantage is not given to one or several providers.
- Follow the EU procurement directives if they apply, but also remember that the EU Treaty principles of equal treatment, transparency, proportionality and free movement of goods apply to all public sector contracts regardless of whether the full EU regulations apply.
- Reduce the cost and time spent on procurement for both purchasers and providers by streamlining the procurement process whenever possible. For example, only ask for relevant information, use framework agreements and e-enabled systems.
- Avoid spot purchasing and instead aggregate spend and seek out opportunities for collaboration. However, be mindful that other service aims such as personalisation are not compromised or that the market is being stifled and choice reduced.
- Make sure that any procurement complies with local financial regulations and/or standing orders.
- Adopt a broad definition of value for money and consider social, environmental and economic issues of relevance to the procurement. Also think about the whole-life cost and do not just consider the initial price.
- Keep a comprehensive record of all the procurement activities undertaken, such as selection decisions and reasons.
- Understand contract law, and be clear about what commitments have been made by the purchaser and the provider and wherever possible use the purchasing organisation's terms and conditions rather than the provider's.

> ## Stop and Reflect
>
> - Are there actions you could take in your organisation to improve procurement and contracting to secure greater benefits?

Summary

This chapter has considered the role of procurement and contracting in the commissioning process and some of the factors that influence decisions to procure services. In summary:

- Procurement is a heavily regulated area and public services are expected to ensure that any processes are open, fair and transparent. The rules and regulations governing this area fall into three main categories: EU procurement directives; national legislation and guidance; and internal organisational processes and polices.
- At a strategic level there are often opportunities to achieve value for money by undertaking procurement activities such as spend analysis and collaborative procurement.
- The contract process consists of 10 steps from 'identifying the requirement' to 'lessons learnt' and forms an integral part of the overall commissioning cycle.
- Commissioners have a key role in the procurement process but need to work closely with their procurement colleagues to ensure that the full benefits of procurement can be utilised and that the process is used to best effect to achieve the desired outcomes.

Further reading and web-based resources

For information regarding the EU procurement directives see http://ec.europa.eu/internal_market/publicprocurement/index_en.htm; details regarding the EU remedies directives are available at http://ec.europa.eu/internal_market/publicprocurement/infringements/remedies/index_en.htm

Information about the EU remedies directives can also be found in the NHS Confederation briefing available from www.nhsconfed.org/Publications/Documents/Euro_Briefing_5_final.pdf

The Local Government Association provides information for elected members and local authority staff on a range of topics including procurement. For further information see their website. www.local.gov.uk/

The Department for Education has published a wide range of information about procurement skills in relation to services for children, young people and families that can be downloaded from www.education.gov.uk/childrenandyoungpeople/strategy/a0065946/procurementskills

Advice for schools on buying goods and services is available from the Department for Education's website at www.education.gov.uk/schools/adminandfinance/procurement

The National Market Development Forum briefing note on Social Care Procurement provides information on procurement, state aid and consultation matters relevant to the provision of social care services and can be downloaded from www.thinklocalactpersonal.org. uk/_library/Resources/Personalisation/Personalisation_advice/2011/23.6.11_SOCIAL_ PROCUREMENT_DOC.pdf

A procurement guide for commissioners of NHS-funded services is available from www. dh.gov.uk/en/Publicationsandstatistics/Publications/PublicationsPolicyAndGuidance/ DH_118218

NCVO and NAVCA have published a guide on procurement specifically aimed at people working for a local charity, voluntary organisation, community group or social enterprise: *Pathways Through the Maze: A Guide to Procurement Law*. Copies can be ordered from www.ncvo-vol.org.uk/pathways

The Office of Government Commerce is now part of the Efficiency and Reform Group within the Cabinet Office. However, a wide range of its previously published guidance can still be accessed from the national archives at http://webarchive.nationalarchives.gov. uk/20110601212617/http:/www.ogc.gov.uk/index.asp.

References

Bevan Brittan (2012) *Public Services (Social Value) Act 2012*. Available at: www.bevanbrittan. com/ARTICLES/Pages/SocialValueAct2012.aspx. Accessed 25 April 2012.

Cook, M., Monk, G. and Reason, J.(eds) (2009) *Pathways Through the Maze: A Guide to Procurement Law*. Sheffield and London: NCVO and NAVCA.

Department for Children, Schools and Families (n.d.) *Procurement Document No 2: Key Principles of Procurement*. Available at: http://media.education.gov.uk/assets/files/doc/k/ key%20principles%20of%20procurement.doc. Accessed 2 May 2012.

Department for Communities and Local Government (2011a) *Best Value Statutory Guidance*. London: DCLG Publications.

Department for Communities and Local Government (2011b) *The Code of Recommended Practice for Local Authorities on Data Transparency*. London: Department for Communities and Local Government.

Department for Education (n.d. a) *Strategic Procurement – An Overview*. Available at: http:// media.education.gov.uk/assets/files/doc/s/strategic%20procurement%20-%20an%20 overview.doc. Accessed 26 April 2012.

Department for Education (n.d. b) *The Contracting Process – An Overview*. Available at: http://media.education.gov.uk/assets/files/doc/t/the%20contracting%20process%20-%20 an%20overview.doc. Accessed 26 April 2012.

Department for Education (2010a) *How To: Apply Category Management to Children's Services*. Available at: http://media.education.gov.uk/assets/files/doc/h/how%20to%20 apply%20category%20management%20to%20childrens%20services.doc. Accessed 26 April 2012.

Department for Education (2010b) *How To: Build Sustainability into Children's Services Procurement*. Available at: http://media.education.gov.uk/assets/files/doc/h/how%20 to%20build%20sustainability%20into%20childrens%20services%20procurement.doc. Accessed 26 April 2012.

Dudkin, G. and Välilä, T. (2005) *Transaction Costs In Public–Private Partnerships: A First Look at the Evidence*, Economic and Financial Report 2005/03. Luxembourg: European Investment Bank.

e-notes (2012) *Make or Buy Decisions.* Available at: www.enotes.com/make-buy-decisions-reference/make-buy-decisions. Accessed 25 May 2012.

Haslam, A. (n.d.) *Benefits of Spend Analysis.* Birmingham: Improvement and Efficiency West Midlands.

HM Government (2011) *Open Public Services White Paper.* London: Cabinet Office.

HM Government (2012a) *Open Public Services 2012.* London: Cabinet Office.

HM Government (2012b) *Public Services (Social Value) Act 2012.* London: TSO.

IDeA (2012) *Procurement and the Equality Act.* Available at: www.idea.gov.uk/idk/core/page.do?pageId=10527774. Accessed 24 February 2012.

Improvement and Efficiency West Midlands (n.d.) *eAuctions: Your Route to Delivering Significant Savings in Procurement Through the Use of eAuctions.* Birmingham: Improvement and Efficiency West Midlands.

National Market Development Forum (2011) *Social Care Procurement.* Available at: www.education.gov.uk/childrenandyoungpeople/strategy/a0065946/procurementskills. Accessed 26 April 2012.

Newton, R. (2011) *Open Public Services White Paper Briefing*, UrbanForum Online. Available at: www.urbanforum.org.uk/briefings/open-public-services-white-paper-briefing. Accessed 24 May 2012.

Office for Government Commerce (2008) *Procurement Guidance: Introduction to EU Procurement Rules.* Norwich: Office for Government Commerce.

10

Contracting for Personalised Services

At the time of writing, commissioners and providers of social care have a range of policy challenges facing them, of which personalisation and the pressure for financial savings and efficiencies are perhaps the greatest. This is partly because the two challenges are potentially contradictory: the economies of scale to be gained from block contracts run directly counter to the delivery of personalised, tailored services aiming to provide choice and control to the individual. In the past, direct provision and block contracts have been seen as an efficient method for local authorities, as they have enabled long term planning with lower transaction costs. Contracting for personalised services involves managing the balance between providing financial flexibility to meet individual needs as and when they arise, while ensuring market stability and sustainability, so that a range of providers enter the market to offer the variety of services required to meet those needs.

Delivering effective personalised services requires changes in the way that commissioners contract with providers for public care. A number of different approaches to contracting have emerged to support the move to personalisation, but understanding of their application, effectiveness and interrelationship remains limited. Most commissioners and providers accept that there is still significant work ahead to develop further, refine, and embed local systems of self-direct support and the infrastructure that underpins them. This chapter looks at the implications of personalisation for contracting and presents the key contractual models which are available. It discusses the effect of personalised contracting on relationships and the implications for commissioners, providers and the wider market.

Learning outcomes

By the end of the chapter you should be able to:

- Define the key concepts and components of a personalised approach to contracting.
- Recognise different models of contracting for personalised services.
- Understand some techniques and methods relating to a person-centred approach.
- Identify some of the implications and potential issues for successful personalised contracting.

Key terms

- *Personal budgets* – a personal budget is money that is available to someone who needs support. The money comes from their local authority social services and is allocated to the individual to spend on help and support to meet their assessed eligible needs.
- *Spot contracts* – these are price-per-case arrangements where prices and other terms are agreed in relation to an individual unit of service, usually around a person receiving care.
- *Block contracts* – Block contracts involve purchasing the total quantity of a service expected to be required over a period of time. Payment is agreed and made in advance, regardless of whether that service is subsequently actually used.

Personalisation

There is a clear government commitment to greater personalisation and choice in health and social care. Personalisation and the wider requirements of the push for public service reform aimed at putting people (users of services) first have been the main drivers for recent contextual changes in contracting practice. The central focus of personalisation is responding to individuals' needs, wants and hopes, rather than fitting people into existing services; and ensuring that they have the means and support to live a full life and contribute to society (English Community Care Association, 2010). To achieve these objectives requires new contracting models and different relationships between those involved.

For both commissioners and providers, personalisation requires a greater focus on choice, flexibility and outcomes. In general, personalisation has been welcomed by providers, for example, the English Community Care Association (2010) states that:

Personalisation presents opportunities for providers to ensure better outcomes for service users and increased opportunities to engage staff, to attract new business and to work more flexibly.

However, there are a number of issues and potential obstacles which we discuss later in the chapter. For example, personalisation implies less local authority purchasing overall and less block contracting. As a result some existing contracted services may become unviable and will need to be downsized or discontinued, in partnership with the people affected and the relevant providers.

The three key components to contracting for personalised services that this chapter will explore are:

- Personal budgets
- Service personalisation
- New contractual models

Personal budgets

Current policy requires that over time, all people with ongoing care and support needs who are eligible for state funding should receive it through a personal budget:

> We will extend the greater roll-out of personal budgets to give people and their carers more control and purchasing power. We will use direct payments to carers and better community-based provision to improve access to respite care. (Department of Health, 2010)

A personal budget can be taken as:

- A direct payment (DP) enabling a service user to purchase their own care which may mean employing staff themselves or contracting with support agencies which employ staff.
- An account held and managed by the public body (LA or NHS) in accordance with individual wishes.
- An Individual Service Fund (ISF) – an account managed by a service provider on behalf of an individual under a council/NHS contract. The money is restricted for use on providing care and support services for that individual which meet the criteria set out in their support plan. It can include services purchased from other providers.
- A combination of direct payments and a managed account.

In addition, some services may continue to be directly purchased by the local authority. Each mechanism has implications for the way in which social care services are specified, tendered and contracted in future.

Figure 10.1 illustrates the difference between contracting for a personalised service with a direct payment, compared with an ISF.

Personal budgets enable choice so long as they are accompanied by the right level of support. An early evaluation found that personal budgets had largely positive outcomes for adults with physical disabilities, people with learning disabilities, and mental health needs, but were less positive for older people who described the 'additional burden' of planning and managing their own support (IBSEN, 2008). Personal

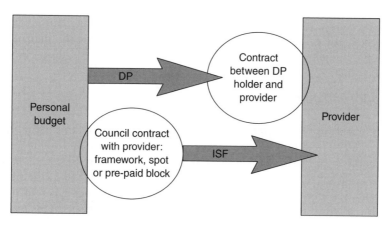

Figure 10.1   ISF, direct payments and contracts

Source: Department of Health, 2009

budgets for disabled children and their families and children with special educational needs (SEN) were piloted in 2011 and, at the time of writing, legislation is proposed (Department for Education, 2012).

Service personalisation

Though some providers have developed and personalised their services independently, most require continuing support to understand the implications of personalisation and to transform their services accordingly. This may involve a significant shift in staff, roles and organisational culture. In particular, support may help them to adapt and personalise their services so that they can provide more flexible services. Some local authorities provide active developmental support to promote more collaborative approaches to commissioning and service development.

The success of a personalised approach to contracting for someone with support needs will be affected by two key components: the degree of choice of service and/or provider that is available to them; and the range and type of support that is available to help them make that choice.

Choice is enhanced when the framework contract can ensure that a good range of providers are available to cover a wide variety of needs, offering services of sufficient quality and a range of options for people regardless of where they live or whether they are state or self-funded. Equally, people should be supported to use providers from outside the framework if they choose. Arrangements for self-funders are also important. In theory, this will mean a better experience for service users and more positive outcomes for them. Personalised contracting focuses on what can be achieved rather than barriers, and promotes dialogue about needs between the service user and providers.

However, contracting for personalised services means that more than a good choice of accessible provision needs to be available to purchasers. Individual purchasers need help to enable them to make the right choices, including affordable services, information about prices, quality, the market, and options for the management of their personal budgets.

Market, price and quality information

Market information is essential for budget holders and good contracting. Knowing which providers can supply what services, and at what price and quality, is important for people with direct payments, commissioners holding ISFs, and self-funders in order to contract for the right services, of the right quality and at the right price. Price information may help to ensure parity between different types of purchaser, although it may limit the scope for tailored, more flexible services. One approach is to set a common 'basic rate' with the option of 'add-ons'.

Budget management options

As personal budgets are due to become the standard model of delivery for all those with ongoing care and support needs, and people will have the choice of a direct payment, local authority managed account or ISF, or a combination of these options, providers and contracts need to be compatible with these various options for managing a personal budget.

In addition, many service users have fluctuating needs which means there is a need for flexibility to vary the amount of personal budget over time, so that service users can vary the volume and type of service provided to meet their needs.

Contractual models

In the past, contracting and purchasing in public care has been dominated by inputs and outputs. Contracts have often only allowed minimal flexibility and limited the discretion of providers to respond to people who use services in the way that best meets their needs. Commissioning for personalised care requires greater flexibility within and between services as well as more effective integration between services than may have previously been the case, particularly in drawing up contracts that define outcomes much more clearly.

The response to the above by many local authorities is to consider a range of new contractual models and new approaches to procurement which are not mutually exclusive:

Framework contracts and approved provider lists

Framework contracts aim to assure quality and supply through pre-selection or validation of providers. Framework contracts do not have to guarantee demand for, or volume of, service and can include some person-centred 'mini-tenders' for people to draw down upon the contracts. Providers included within a framework contract can be required to deliver services in more flexible and personalised ways regardless of whether or not their customers are self- or state-funded. Here, in effect, the local authority is giving a 'seal of approval' to one or more providers, but leaves the service user free to select who they might use.

Most authorities have adopted a framework approach to contracting for domiciliary care. This has involved providers signing up to provide flexible and personalised services without a minimum guarantee of volume or demand. The detail of the service delivered to an individual is determined between the personal budget holder and the provider, based on information in their support plan, though the framework identifies broad outcomes for the contract overall. To ensure accessibility and the extension of choice and control to a wider range of people, frameworks can also require providers to make ISFs (or their equivalent by another name) available to personal budget holders.

Framework contracts and approved provider lists allow a way for people who opt for the local authority to manage their personal budget to draw on a range of 'approved' services. It is important that people have the information, support and guidance to purchase services outside these contracts if they wish; with a clear understanding of any implications, risks and benefits. The local authority's contracting practice should not unnecessarily restrict the choices available to those who cannot manage or do not opt for a direct payment.

In 2009, the Department of Health considered the way that domiciliary care contracts were changing across six local authority areas, which already had high numbers of personal budget holders, and were preparing for further expansion.

> ... all but one of the sites has adopted a framework approach to contracting for domiciliary care. This has involved providers signing up to provide flexible and personalised services without a minimum guarantee of volume or demand. In all cases, the detail of the service delivered to an individual is determined between the personal budget holder and the provider based on information in their support plan, though the framework identifies broad outcomes for the contract overall. To ensure accessibility and the extension of choice and control to a wider range of people, the frameworks have also required providers to make ISFs (or their equivalent by another name) available to personal budget holders. (Department of Health, 2009)

Individual Service Funds (ISFs)

ISFs offer a way for personal budget holders who choose not to direct some or all of their support through direct payments to manage their money. The local authority transfers the personal budget to a provider (or sub contractor) on an individual's behalf ensuring the individual has maximum control over any support provided; and the individual is empowered to work with the provider to decide the exact detail of any support provided, for example, the timing and the tasks to be carried out. As part of a framework contract, councils can include a requirement that providers make ISFs available to their clients.

Mini-tenders

Some authorities use 'mini-tendering' to determine which provider from within the framework contract will offer support to an individual or group of individuals. This anonymised information from individual support plans, along with confirmation of the indicative budget, is sent to providers who are encouraged to respond to the mini-tender with a plan for how they will support the person or persons. People and families remain involved throughout the process, evaluating bids and determining which provider will deliver the support.

Outcome-based contracts

The service user and the local authority agree the outcomes to be achieved and a given price. The service user and provider negotiate over when services are required and how they are to be delivered in order to achieve the specified outcomes. A broker or the local authority is available in the case of disputes. Outcome-focused contracts help commissioners to concentrate on what they want the provider to achieve and why, rather than the volume of service provided. Achieving outcomes can be both collectively and individually more motivating than providing an amount of service, while raising quality and potentially enhancing working relationships.

Guarantee contracts

The local authority agrees with a provider to underwrite a given volume of service purchase at an agreed price.

Fixed price procurement

The value of the contract is given together with an assessment of how that market price has been determined. Providers bid against what they can offer for the price.

Aggregated contracts

A group of personal budget holders get together, with or without the help of the local authority, in order to purchase a set of common services.

There are a number of circumstances where competitive tendering and block contracts remain appropriate. For example, in the case of the former then tendering may be appropriate where:

- Entirely new services are needed.
- A high cost/volume of services is being purchased on behalf of users by the local authority.
- There has been a challenge to the fairness of existing procurement practices.
- Current services have consistently failed to respond to need.
- Costs of services are considered unacceptably high or unjustified.

On the other hand, there may be circumstances where negotiations with current providers can achieve the same outcome, or where direct feedback from service users and carers can help to secure the improvements needed. In areas where services are hard to procure or develop, then pump priming funding or premium payments may be needed in order to ensure availability.

In terms of block contracts, it is important to recognise that delivering the 'choice' element of choice and control is not necessarily just about a choice of provider.

Choice can equally entail a choice of services being available from one provider, or the timing of service delivery, or who the care worker is. There may be circumstances where block or guaranteed contracts may be the best way of achieving these elements of choice. However, where this approach is to be used, service users need to play a part in all aspects of the process. For the local authority, building up the capacity of service users to contribute, steer or even control the tendering process is crucial. For providers, services which are genuinely user-led are likely to be able to show that their approach and design will best meet the needs of purchasers in the future. This may also mean the local authority going beyond the 'usual suspects' or organisations in getting genuine service user representation.

A new management team in a shire county decided to make a radical overhaul of their contracting arrangements for home care in order to move to a personalised, outcomes-based approach. They decided to contract for a service built around the expressed wishes of service users to provide integrated help for people to live at home, including equipment, telecare and the out of hours response service.

At least six meetings took place between potential providers and the commissioning team before the formal tendering process. Eight outcome-focused contracts were awarded to four different providers. Providers were allocated a sum of money based on the defined outcomes that the service user and their assessment and care management worker agreed. The provider was responsible with the customer for the delivery of these outcomes. Everyone was offered an initial support plan, regardless of their means.

The initiative has required commissioners, assessment and care management, providers and carers to all change their current practices. After initial scepticism, staff warmed to the approach as the process is quicker and gives users a stronger voice. Providers have welcomed improved information sharing with the commissioner and it is expected that the approach will reduce costs over time.

CASE STUDY

(continued)

(continued)

A key lesson has been that if a local authority wishes to move to personalised outcomes-based contracting arrangements, it needs to transform both its care management and contracting systems. The commissioning team found that transforming contracting has taken time (three years), and it was critical to engage all key stakeholders including providers at all stages of the contracting process in order to get the final shape of the service right.

Interrelationships

Figure 10.2 illustrates the interrelationship between personalised services, personal budgets and a framework contract. The 'professionally controlled' options on the left hand side contrast with those on the right that are 'personalised'. The 'professionally controlled' options, even when allocating personalised services, are not fully aligned to personalisation, as they do not give the person requiring support a choice of which provider to use or what kind of support is provided. In theory, over time, the unshaded areas should become obsolete as people move across to personalised contracting.

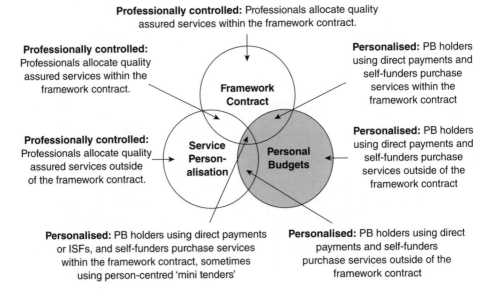

Figure 10.2   Interrelationship diagram

Source: Department of Health, 2009

Local authority contracting

Notwithstanding personalisation, there is likely to be a continued role for the local authority in purchasing some people's care and support. This may be via a range of framework agreements or where the local authority part purchases the core elements of certain services, with the user choosing and/or purchasing the remaining elements of their care. Circumstances in which local authorities still need to retain or even develop their contracting role include:

- Where the local authority can bring its purchasing power to bear for service users who opt for services purchased in this way and arranged by the local authority;
- Where an existing relationship with a provider needs to be supported but individualised;
- Where certain specialist services are required, particularly 'mixed packages' with the NHS, for example to treat and provide security for people with mental health or other conditions;
- Where people wishing to purchase support, particularly those wanting to employ Personal Assistants, need the availability and access to specialist support, for example to assist with recruitment, payroll, insurance and tax (Scottish Government, 2009).

Stop and Reflect

In contracting for personalised services, you need to think about who purchases, and increasingly the nature of the purchase decision itself. Figure 10.3 presents the three key questions to consider when you are involved in contracting arrangements:

- Who is purchasing?
- What is the basis of the contract?
- What factors are likely to be key drivers behind the process?

The answers will depend on the context you are working in and what contracting model is in operation. How well are your arrangements working? Is there more you could do to enable personal budget holders to make good choices?

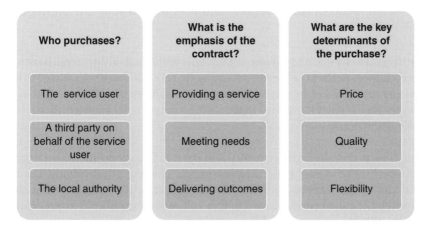

Figure 10.3   Key decisions

How does contracting for personalised services affect relationships between those involved?

There are very different views about how procurement and contracting relationships and behaviours will develop with the personalisation of social care. Some writers suggest the likelihood of an increasingly adversarial culture in the market:

> The procurement landscape is changing with an ever increasing number of challenges to procurement processes .... Bid costs and accountability are more important than ever in the current economic climate .... Bidders are now entitled to significantly more information that may alert them to potential breaches of the regulations. More crucially bidders may face damaging exclusion from a market if unsuccessful in a procurement. Failure to be awarded a contract or be included on a framework can be potentially devastating for a business. (Gilliam and Heatley, 2010)

Others suggest that this may be less of an issue, as tendering and contracting will become more person-centred, and block contracting and associated competitive tendering will reduce:

> Personalisation means that where commissioners continue to play a direct role in specifying and procuring services, there will be a strategic shift away from task- and time-based (tendering) towards outcomes-focused and person-centred approaches. This may include a reduction in block contracting for many services as these can reduce the choice available to people ... New contractual models that support the move to personalisation include framework contracts and approved provider lists – where people opting for the council to manage their personal budget can draw upon a range of 'approved' services. (SCIE, 2009)

Others suggest that placing an emphasis on tendering activities which improve the balance of risk between commissioners and providers to stimulate greater innovation will be important:

> Everything carries a risk, and failures already exist within publicly delivered health and social care. There needs to be greater willingness to take calculated risks related to innovation and new forms of delivery, while ensuring it is shared between both parties and that excessive risk is not transferred to social enterprises or other providers. (Social Enterprise Coalition, 2008)

Another view is that the local authority will need to change its focus, perhaps away from competitive tendering altogether, leaving purchasing to individuals. The role of the local authority will be as an influencer through effective signalling of likely need and of purchasing intentions. However, this will require significant improvements in the quality of information available to all parties:

... councils were not good at signalling their purchasing intentions in the short term, nor did they signal the need for new services ... they did not signal the services that might be needed in the long term, regardless of the numbers of people the council might support financially. In some instances, where councils did have discussions about future intentions, particularly about the development of new services, the private sector was often excluded (or perceived itself to be). (CSCI, 2007)

The impact of the changes in the contracting and procurement landscape on relationships between local authorities and providers depends, at least in part, on whether they choose to work collaboratively or adversarially.

New tendering processes need to reflect changes in the relationships between the local authority, the provider and individual service users/carers that will result from the personalisation agenda. For example this may mean moving from:

- The local authority as a sole purchaser, to one where providers will need to market to (and contract with) a larger number of individual service purchasers.
- Large block contracts to individual service contracts and arrangements, although perhaps underpinned by a framework agreement between the local authority and one or more providers.
- Formal structured arrangements for the procurement and delivery of social care to a more flexible approach where achieving agreed outcomes for a given price is the contractual focus rather than the volume or nature of service delivered.

Figure 10.4 presents the traditional relationship between the service user, the local authority and the service provider. The local authority assesses need, allocates resources and procures a service from the provider. The service user is a passive recipient of the service which has been procured for them.

Figure 10.5 presents a picture of how relationships may develop in the future with the service user taking a more active role: identifying their needs, specifying and securing services directly from the provider and feeding back on performance. Meanwhile the local authority retains a residual role in agreeing assessments, service plans and outcomes, but develops a greater role in facilitating the market and promoting community organisations. All three parties are engaged in using and sharing information, managing resources, and monitoring achievements and outcomes.

In exploring new or changed relationships to the procurement process there are challenges at both an individual, as well as at a wider market level. For example, each party in Figure 10.5 planning to contract for a specific service may have different priorities in terms of:

- Price
- Quality
- Risk and safety
- Control
- Flexibility and reliability

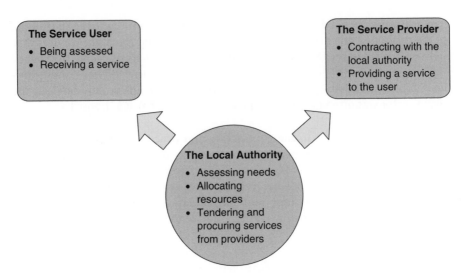

Figure 10.4   Traditional relationships

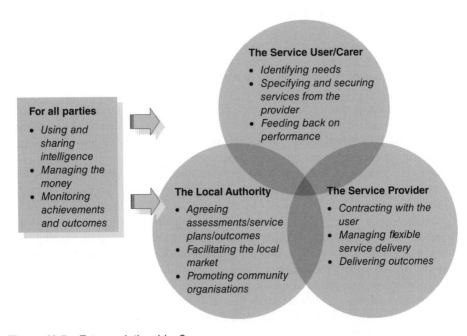

Figure 10.5   Future relationships?

This requires negotiation and will be easier where good relationships between those concerned are well established.

> ## Stop and Reflect
>
> - What kind of relationship do you have with provider organisations and service users?
> - What active steps are you taking to develop and maintain good relationships?
> - Do you understand what their priorities are?
> - Can you build on areas of common interest?

Implications for commissioners and providers

The introduction of contracting for personalised services has implications for commissioners and providers. Some are shared and some are specific to one or the other.

Moving from existing block contracts

The shift from block contracts involves a whole system change for both parties in terms of planning, delivery, invoicing and payment for services. Commissioners can help providers by signalling to them ahead of time where they are planning to move to a personalised contracting model, for example, with a market position statement (see Chapter 8). They can also help them to prepare partly through sharing information, but also by discussing tapering arrangements: extending block contracts for a while to enable providers to adapt to the new market or phasing them out gradually as demand for ISFs grows. Encouraging flexibility of provision may be a key part of the local authority commissioning role in the future.

Managing potential 'transitional' demand and supply issues

Local authorities differ in the degree to which their services are spot bought or block contracted, and hence how quickly they can move away from providers who do not wish to enter into new contractual arrangements. Good relationships with providers can be key to implementing changes within existing contracts. Inevitably, moving to new contracts does involve some decommissioning from providers who do not wish to offer more personalised services, or whose services are not of sufficient quality (see Chapter 12).

Supply side adjustments

Personalisation may involve supply side adjustments by providers to meet service user demand. Providers will need to consider the stability of their income streams in an environment where block contracting arrangements with commissioners are replaced by spot contracting arrangements with individuals. Collaboration with other providers may enable them to maximise opportunities for service delivery to individuals. Providers will also need to consider the effect of consumer legislation when contracting with individuals.

A range of research also suggests that flexibility in terms of what care and support is delivered and when, is of concern to the whole market of service users. Providers have to be more flexible than they have been in the past, in order to adjust to fluctuations in user demand for services as their needs vary and change. This is particularly challenging for those services where small changes in the level of demand may affect the sustainability of the business, such as small providers for whom losing one contract represents a significant proportion of their total business. Some providers will have to change their accounting and financial management systems to enable them to charge on an individual basis.

Recruitment and training

In addition, a move to contracting for personalised services may require recruitment and training of new and existing staff to work in a more personalised way. For example, staff may need to develop better customer service and marketing skills to attract and maintain clients with personal budgets. There may be scope to pool resources for training staff to deliver personalised services.

Cultural change in all parts of the system

Accompanying systemic changes is the need for cultural change with providers needing to work alongside service users in a more empowering way, embracing the philosophy of 'nothing about me without me' and focusing on enabling people to meet their outcomes, rather than on inputs and outputs. Commissioners also need a more empowering approach focused on identifying what outcomes individuals want to achieve and facilitating the market to deliver them. This means developing a greater understanding of how to enable people to access universal and mainstream services such as housing, leisure and transport; and making more creative use of community capacity such as neighbourhood groups and clubs.

Whether or not service users and carers have direct payments, the implementation of a personalised approach to contracting changes the relationship between professionals and service users, with greater scope for co-production of services and empowerment: working with people, not for them. The emphasis is on empowering personal budget holders and supporting citizens to shape the market for themselves.

Good accessible information

In order to ensure that service users can make informed choices, providers must provide good accessible information about their services in terms of description, cost and quality. Ensuring that accessible information is readily available contributes to effective marketing and quality assurance.

Wider market issues

At the wider market level, whilst many authorities are responding by moving to the new concept of framework agreements, there are still a number of issues to be tackled.

- Moving from a single to a large number of purchasers potentially drives up transaction costs for providers. If local authorities face falling budgets, paying a higher price for the same provision may not be a viable option.
- In many instances the local authority may still remain a significant purchaser, buying on behalf of service users who do not wish or are not able to act as purchasers in their own right. In these circumstances what makes for the best purchasing arrangements?
- Some providers will be concerned about market destabilisation if the certainty of block contracts is removed. Particularly for smaller providers, managing a diverse set of arrangements combined with uncertainty about take up, may drive them out of business.
- Some providers may see framework agreements as providing all the difficulties and costs associated with traditional tendering but with the added disadvantage that there is no guarantee of customers at the end of the process.
- Providers may feel added pressure if they are bidding to deliver a regulated care service with a trained workforce but having to compete against unregulated care in the form of personal assistants.
- If there is a greater emphasis on the marketing of care services to both self-funders and those with personal budgets, then smaller providers may lose out as their capacity to market their provision may not be as great as that of larger providers.

Employment issues

There are a number of responsibilities and risks where a provider is directly employed by a service user, either using their personal budget or as a self-funder. These have been identified by the Association of Chief Executives of Voluntary Organisations (ACEVO) as:

- Statutory obligations: working time regulations; managing a payroll; statutory guidelines around hazardous work; statutory guidelines around night work; statutory guidelines around rest breaks.
- Some considerations on annual leave: all employees will be eligible for statutory holiday; atypical workers, e.g. shift workers, casual workers, part-time workers, will have different holiday allowances.

- The user will have to carry public liability and employer's liability insurance.
- The following pre-employment checks will need to be carried out: health checks; references; qualifications; Independent Safeguarding Authority (ISA); Criminal Records Bureau (CRB).
- Income tax and NI will have to be applied.
- Health and safety obligations will have to be performed, including: risk analysis for those using machinery and equipment, driving, lifting and carrying or working in awkward spaces.
- Personal data will have to be safeguarded.
- Fair, non-discriminatory employment practices will have to be followed. (ACEVO, 2010)

Service users concerns

Some service users and their families may be apprehensive about the move to a personalised approach. This may be due to a concern about new responsibilities, anxiety that it could result in a decline in service quality, and a general resistance to change in long-standing arrangements. It is important to ensure that service users and carers understand what is involved and are supported to make the choices appropriate to their needs. The choices that matter to service users may be about who will be their key worker, rather than which organisation provides the service.

Stop and Reflect

- What are the challenges of personalisation for your organisation? For example, do you have sufficient resources, information on quality and cost, and a wide range of good quality providers?
- What services does the local authority need to continue to purchase directly?
- What are the concerns of service users locally and how are you addressing them?

Legal aspects – risk and safeguarding

Those involved in the contracting process need to be mindful of the specific issues and potential barriers relating to the creation of new services, such as cash flow, entry and transaction costs, regulatory compliance, employment law and complex procurement procedures (see Chapter 9).

The legal framework surrounding the personalisation agenda is still unclear. Very little public law and almost no case law means that, although there are currently government targets for personal budgets, there is little understanding of the legal implications of implementing them. There are questions about what legal safeguards exist for service users employing personal assistants (PAs) and, equally, how the rights of support workers and carers employed by individuals can be protected.

Direct payments can be paid to a 'user representative' if the service user lacks capacity, but issues can arise in relation to user representatives' liability in this context. A service user can accept aspects of the care plan and the risks involved as long as he/she understands the risk, i.e. has capacity. Service users should therefore be educated about risks.

Commissioning public bodies continue to have a responsibility to monitor risk under both statutory and common law. For example, local authorities have a responsibility to ensure that services that they commission promote the welfare and safeguarding of children (DCSF, 2010). Service providers should work with their commissioners to use multi-agency procedures when concerns arise regarding safeguarding of vulnerable people or children.

There are risk assessment issues when an individual's capacity to make decisions is impaired and an agency manages their personal budget (ISF) for them (e.g. brokers, or in some cases service providers). It raises questions about who should make such decisions: the service user, the family or professional health and care staff? These issues are equally applicable to those using their own money (i.e. self-funders) as personal budget-holders, and there is likely to be an ongoing tension between safety and risk, and the competency of the individual to make those decisions.

Regulation

It is important to ensure that the approach adopted by regulators encourages personalised commissioning, for example, by checking that its underpinning values find expression in agreed standards, and that registered services therefore in turn reflect these values. It is also important that inspectors are assisted to understand both the spirit and the letter of such improved standards. This is crucial within a system of personalised contracting, and commissioners are required to take account of and accept the findings of regulation and inspection.

There are particular issues relating to whether purchasing by people with direct payments should be regulated for quality, safety and value for money in the same way as for other provision. The process of regulation may need to be reviewed when personalised contracting and individual budgets become the norm for people using social care services, and as the number of direct payment recipients increases. Many of the arguments have already been rehearsed with the initial development of direct payments.

The wider argument is about the validity of people's choices, and about when public money ceases to be 'public' with a corresponding reduction in the level of monitoring and accountability for expenditure required. A narrower issue is whether people who employ their own personal assistant are subject to the same obligations as agencies in relation to making safe recruitment checks and meeting other social service employer requirements. As social care registration extends to wider groups of home care and support staff, with all of the attendant training and qualification requirements, there could be similar issues about whether personal assistant employers may only employ registered staff.

A number of potential obstacles to successful contracting for personalised services have been identified. How might you address the following within your organisation using the information in this chapter?

- Fear of change and an aversion to risk
- Dominance of interest groups that want to maintain the status quo
- Staff trained to work in the system, not towards outcomes for people
- Reluctance to accept that services may have to be decommissioned
- Lack of flexibility to respond to what people want, beyond specifications
- Lack of information – about what people's needs and preferences are
- Lack of information – for people about possibilities and choices
- Poor relationships within the public sector, with differing priorities
- Rigid processes, e.g. inflexible block contracts or service specifications
- Adversarial, legalistic relationships between commissioners and providers
- Lack of focus on outcomes for people

Summary

This chapter sets out the key elements of contracting for personalised services, the new contractual models which have emerged in response to the personalisation agenda and the implications of this approach. Contracting for personalised services involves a system-wide change affecting commissioners, providers, service users and carers. The aim is to empower and enable those receiving services to achieve the outcomes they desire.

Further reading and web-based resources

Department of Health (2009) *Putting People First Programme Contracting for Personalised Outcomes: Learning from Emerging Practice.* London: HMSO.
Scottish Government (2009) *A Personalised Commissioning Approach to Support and Care Services,* Changing Lives Service Development Group. Edinburgh: Scottish Government.
www.in-control.org.uk/publications/reports-and-discussion-papers/briefing-1-personalisation-children,-young-people-and-families.aspx

References

ACEVO (2010) *Personalisation: Exploring the Legal Implications.* London: ACEVO.
CSCI (2007) *Safe as Houses? What Drives Investment in Social Care?* London: CSCI.

Department for Children, Schools and Families (2010) *Working Together to Safeguard Children: A Guide to Inter-agency Working to Safeguard and Promote the Welfare of Children,* London: HMSO. Available at: http://publications.dcsf.gov.uk/default.aspx?Page Function=productdetails&PageMode=publications&ProductId=DCSF-00305-2010

Department for Education (2012) *Support and Aspiration: A New Approach to Special Educational Needs and Disability – Progress and Next Steps.* London: HMSO.

Department of Health (2009) *Contracting for Personalised Outcomes: Learning from Emerging Practice,* Putting People First Programme. London: HMSO.

Department of Health (2010) *A Vision for Adult Social Care: Capable Communities and Active Citizens.* London: HMSO.

English Community Care Association (2010) *Personalising Care: A Route Map to Delivery for Care Providers.* London: The Care Provider Alliance.

Gilliam, B. and Heatley, L. (2010) in *Community Care Market News,* May.

IBSEN (2008) *Evaluation of the Individual Budgets Pilot Programme: Final Report.* York: SPRU.

SCIE (2009) *Personalisation Briefing: Implications for Commissioners.* London: SCIE.

Scottish Government (2009) *A Personalised Commissioning Approach to Support and Care Services,* Changing Lives Service Development Group. Edinburgh: Scottish Government.

Social Enterprise Coalition (2008) *Healthy Business: A Guide to Social Enterprise in Health and Social Care.* London: Hempsons; Social Enterprise Coalition.

Section 4

Review

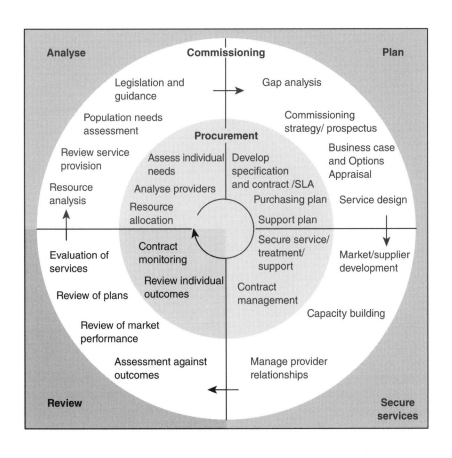

11

Managing Service Performance

One of the key messages in this book is that commissioning has to be clear and purposeful. Councils and other public sector commissioners want to ensure that services are available that will meet local needs and commissioning is an important tool for any agency in achieving its objectives for public care.

We anticipate for example that Local Authorities will be commissioning services to keep families safe and to reduce admissions to residential care where they can. For older people and younger adults commissioners will want to ensure that the services available will help to promote independence and wellbeing. It is therefore important that public care bodies have a set of measures in place which can be used to establish whether they are achieving the objectives which they have set.

Performance management is a term which refers to the different levels of measuring performance that need to be achieved by an organisation in coming to a view as to whether it is meeting its stated objectives and outcomes. These include:

- The overall performance of the organisation and its key partners in meeting shared objectives.
- The performance of particular parts of the service in meeting specified objectives.
- The performance of individuals within each service area in making their contribution to meeting overall objectives.

Of course it is not commissioners alone who impact on these – there will be other critical groups, such as assessment and care management staff, who will influence what happens. So performance management is an approach which the whole organisation needs to adopt. Measuring performance is vital but the benefits only truly accrue when there is a consistent culture throughout the organisation.

In this chapter the traditional approach to performance management will be examined but with a fresh look at its relevance to the market facilitation role of commissioners and the 'new world' of outcome-based contracting. In addition the importance of relationships between commissioners, providers and users of services will be emphasised for the sustainability of effective performance management.

Learning outcomes

By the end of this chapter you should be able to:

- Apply performance management principles and techniques in commissioning situations.
- Design performance management systems with appropriate measures and outcomes.
- Understand the role of performance management relevant to market place relationships.

Key terms

- *Objective* – what you want to achieve.
- *Performance measures* and *performance indicators* – both used to refer to measures of how well a service is performing against its objectives. SMART measures refer to those that are Specific, Measurable, Achievable, Realistic and Time bounded.
- *Targets* – express a specific level of performance the organisation is aiming to achieve.
- *Standards* – express the minimum acceptable level of performance, or the level of performance that is generally expected.
- *Performance information system* – refers to a set of performance measures for an organisation and the processes for producing that information.
- *Outcomes* – specific changes in behaviour, condition and satisfaction for the people that are served by a project or a service. These gains generally signal improvements or 'human gains' that have been brought about by the service intervention (Centre for Public Innovation).

The benefits of effective PM

The benefits of effective performance management can be summarised as:

- A better understanding of the long term impact of resources in meeting the needs of patients, service users and the population.
- Better understanding of the activities that are taking place, and wheather they are having an impact.

- An opportunity to understand the reasons behind past performance and what needs to change in the future.
- An opportunity to stimulate innovation among providers and incentivise performance.

In short, commissioners need good quality performance information and analysis to help them judge the efficiency and effectiveness of services. Measuring performance is the foundation for good decision making by the commissioner.

Why measure performance?

Measuring the performance of commissioned services helps to ensure that commissioners can:

- Ensure that what gets measured gets done.
- Distinguish between success and failure.
- Identify success and reward it.
- Identify success and replicate it.
- Identify failure and correct it.
- Demonstrate results and win public support.
- Be accountable to the public for taxpayers' spend on public services.

The process of performance measurement is not an end in itself, although it can help organisations improve services. Commisioners need to develop systems that monitor outputs, finances and, crucially, quality and experience of service (including customer feedback) in order to be able to make a judgement about the extent to which services are meeting their requirements and achieving the outcomes desired for individuals, and for the population as a whole.

The key elements of a performance management framework

The key elements of any performance management framework is outlined in Figure 11.1. It includes having clear objectives for services, developing SMART measures and undertaking monitoring of providers; reporting; and taking action on analysed findings.

With in this stage it is worth remembering that:

- Performance Measurement is about defining objectives and measures (or indicators), which should be set out in specification or contracts.
- Performance Monitoring is concerned with what happens after a set of indicators has been defined.

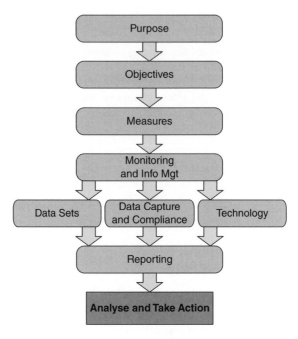

Figure 11.1   The Performance Management model

- Information management is concerned with what data set is to be captured and how to capture it.
- Technology helps to deliver the information needed by commissioners but it is no substitute for commissioners being clear about what they want to measure. There is a tendency to rely on the technology – it should not be the tail wagging the dog.
- Once the information has been captured it then needs to be analysed and reported to be of use (a corrective action plan) – taking action on information is the most important thing.

Measuring outcomes

However, having a good overall framework in place does not inevitably lead to a successful performance management approach in practice. Just as important, within the framework, is being clear about *what* you are measuring and monitoring. The focus on designing and measuring services around outcomes has been a strong theme of commissioning practice over the past few years. One particular exponent has been Mark Friedman in his approach of Outcome/Results Based Accountability (OBA) (Friedman, 2005).

> Results based accountability starts with ends and works back to means. Results-based accountability is a different way of thinking. It organizes the work of programs, agencies,

communities, cities, counties and states around the end conditions we seek for those who live in our community. It uses these end conditions as the grounding for all of the work, including decision making and budgeting.

To illustrate, in Table 11.2 three simple performance measurement categories are given:

- How much service did we deliver – quantity of effort?
- How well did we deliver it – quality of effort?
- Is anyone better off – this covers both bottom quadrants of quantity of effect, i.e. how many service users are better off, and quality of effect, i.e. how are they better off?

The upper left hand quadrant in Table 11.2 is typically the number of service users and activities, e.g. number of residential care places in the local market. This is the easiest to measure quadrant. The upper right quadrant includes measures such as turnover rate and unit cost or service user satisfaction as well as activity-specific measures such as percentage of actions completed on time, percentage of actions meeting standards, or percentage of service users completing activity, e.g. Ofsted rating and cost of residential care settings.

The lower quadrants are to do with the results or outcomes that we want to achieve, for example the number and percentage of young people who stopped using alcohol and drugs or the outcomes for children in residential care. We have least control over the most important measures. It is harder to get data for the lower right hand quadrant, which is why people often focus on the top left quadrant.

Effective performance management means ensuring a balance of measures across the quadrants. It is this balance of measures that need to be represented in the contracting process but with a very specific focus and prominence on outcomes.

Table 11.1 Examples of outcomes, outputs, inputs and processes

Objective	Type
Increase the number of vulnerable adults helped to live in the community	Output
Reduce the number of delayed discharges by 10% over the next 12 months	Output
All new schemes started in 2004/05 to have follow up customer satisfaction surveys during 2005/06	Process
More service users will receive quicker and fairer access to services	Outcome
All staff will be trained and made aware of their responsibilities to protect vulnerable adults from abuse.	Input
Write and agree a protocol for joint working by September 2005	Process
Build a workforce that reflects diversity of the population and which is better supported and trained to meet clients' needs.	Outcome

Table 11.2 OBA measures

How much did we do?	How well did we do it?
# Customers served (by customer characteristic)	% Common measures Workload ratio, staff turnover rate, staff morale, percent of staff fully trained, worker safety, unit cost, customer satisfaction: *Did we treat you well?*
# Activities (by type of activity)	% Activity-specific measures Per cent of actions timely and correct, per cent of clients completing activity, per cent of actions meeting standards
Is Anyone Better Off?	
# **Skills/Knowledge**	% **Skills/Knowledge**
# **Attitude/Opinion**	% **Attitude/Opinion** including customer satisfaction: *Did we help you with your problems?*
# **Behaviour**	% **Behaviour**
# **Circumstance**	% **Circumstance**

Source: Schematic of Outcomes-Based Accountability ™(OBA) performance measures used with permission from the book *Trying Hard is Not Good Enough: How to Produce Measurable Improvements for Customers and Communities,* Mark Friedman (2005).

Stop and Reflect

Effective performance monitoring tips:

- Adopt proportional investment in monitoring with levels of action based on risk
- Collate information from contract monitoring with other sources
- Make use of providers' Quality Assurance systems
- Agree protocols on intervention with underperforming providers
- Set up systems to ensure action is taken
- Publicise performance against standards

Outcome-based contracting

For the commissioner the importance of measuring outcomes needs to be translated into the contracting process. As outcome measurement can be difficult and some outcomes are often out of the control of the provider, a purely outcome-based approach may be only applicable in the minority of cases. A practical approach can be to have a mixture of types of measure (outcomes, outputs, inputs and processes) – but the starting point is to agree the outcomes first then work out what this will mean for practice and measurement.

Table 11.3 illustrates the measures adopted in a contract specification for care support in a supported housing scheme from an IPC client authority. In this example one of the outcomes required for residents was an improvement in daily living (column 1). Six measures were then identified for this outcome as were methodologies to gather the data. It is worth noting that half of these measures are based on the perceptions of the residents themselves.

From a commissioning and contracting perspective, the commissioner needs to be clear how outcomes will be measured and agree methods of verification with the provider. It is necessary to think about how this will be written within the specification and how explicit.

Table 11.3   Measurement framework for outcomes example

Individual outcome	Measures	Methodology
a. On-going improvement, maintenance or minimised deterioration in ability to undertake daily living functions	i. % of residents who perceive that their ability to undertake a daily living function has continued to improve since entering the scheme, e.g. cooking, caring for their own home	Self-assessment/ assisted assessment via discussion
	ii. % reduction in the number of hours/visits attending to residents daily living outcomes	Service provider records, residents' files
	iii. % of residents who perceive that their ability to undertake a daily living function has been maintained since entering the scheme, e.g. cooking, caring for their own home	
	iv. % of residents for whom their number of hours/visits attending to their daily living outcomes has been maintained	
	v. % of residents who perceive that their ability to undertake a daily living function has deteriorated since entering the scheme, e.g. cooking, caring for their own home	
	vi. % of residents for whom their number of hours/visits attending to their daily living outcomes has increased	

Measuring outcomes at the three levels

Performance management frameworks can be applied at three levels to monitor the impact of services and analyse the extent to which they have achieved the purpose intended.

Individual level

The purpose of performance management at individual level is to ensure goods and services are meeting the 'needs' of users. A service may be generally performing well and the contract monitoring process may evidence contract compliance, but it may still be failing to meet an individual's needs. In individual service reviews/feedback, the emphasis should be on whether or not a service is meeting the needs and specified outcomes for the individual user, and appropriate action taken if there are problems.

Operational level

The purpose of performance management at this level is to ensure goods and services are accessible and efficient and are delivering the outcomes appropriate to users' needs. Performance management is about monitoring performance against outcome measures and/or targets, identifying opportunities for improvement and delivering change. Commissioning organisations should develop a clear performance management process which ensures appropriate standards of goods and services are met. However, it should be noted that standards do not always measure outcomes, for example, a person may be receiving really good quality residential care but the outcome should have been to prepare them for independence which has not been achieved.

Strategic level

The purpose of this stage is to ensure the overall shape and performance of goods and services are delivering the required strategic outcomes for the commissioning organisation.

A strategic approach is one that addresses two fundamental questions – are citizens receiving the goods and services they need? Specifically, to what extent are services across the public, private and third sectors configured in the ways intended in the commissioning plan and are further changes needed? In addition what impact are goods and services having on meeting the various outcome needs of the population, and does this need to change?

Examples of measuring performance at the three levels are described below:

Individual level example – the Outcomes Star

Triangle Consulting (2006) have developed a flexible tool for measuring progress of outcomes at an individual level for service users, called the Outcomes Star. Figure 11.2 shows an example which measures the progress for service users receiving support to maximise independence and achieve other goals.

There are different versions of the star including: mental health; homelessness; sexual health; community and an older people's star. All the versions follow a similar pattern consisting of scales and a star chart. This is very much suited to the measuring of aspects of personalisation and can take a much more holistic approach to progress for individuals over time. For example the 'Recovery Star' in Figure 11.2 has been developed for people with mental health problems.

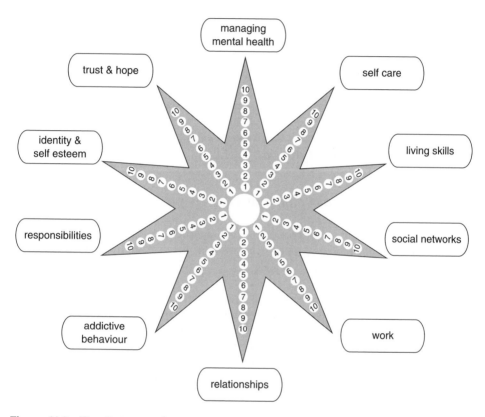

Figure 11.2   The Outcomes Star

The outcome areas focused on within this model are:

- Managing mental health.
- Self care.
- Living skills.
- Social networks.
- Work.
- Relationships.
- Addictive behaviour.
- Responsibilities.
- Identify and self-esteem.
- Trust and hope.

Within each of these areas there is a ladder to help users/families/carers work out where a service user is within that area of their life. These ladders represent stages of change against which the user can assess the current situation for different areas of their life. There are five stages: Stuck (1–2); Accepting help (3–4); Believing (5–6); Learning (7–8); Self-reliance (9–10).

Each star has detailed questions associated with each of these five stages to help gauge where the user is on the ladder for each outcome area. Each step on the ladder is associated with a numerical score (1–10) which can then be plotted onto the star model.

A reading is taken by the worker and service user at the beginning as a baseline measure before intervention, then the process is repeated at regular intervals to track progress and see if outcomes are being achieved.

What this staged approach also offers is the potential to tailor services to where the individual is on the ladder to enable them to move up the ladder, the assumption being that someone who is stuck will require a different intervention to someone who is at the learning stage of change.

Operational level – contract monitoring and review

Achieving outcomes at an operational level is crucial because it is through the mechanism of contracts and specifications for services that so much care is commissioned:

> At the most basic level, managing service performance involves monitoring achievement of the contracted service outputs, ensuring appropriate payment deductions are made, and ensuring that contractual performance improvement processes are enacted and complied with to return performance to the required level, i.e. ensure the local authority is getting what it pays for and also the level of service it has specified. It should also ensure that the service provider is operating in a safe manner in compliance with the appropriate statutes, regulations and policies.

This quote from the Public Private Partnerships Programme (2007) gives the basic focus of contract monitoring and review but specifically the commissioner has four key questions as illustrated in Table 11.4.

In terms of monitoring, the commissioner/provider has to decide what evidence is needed to establish if the outcomes have been met. The categories of evidence and method of data collection will depend on the outcome to be achieved but are broadly illustrated in Figure 11.3. In terms of categories of evidence for outcomes there are two main types:

- Objective evidence – this is the quantitative evidence, specific criteria that demonstrate that there has been change for the individual.
- Perceptions – this is the qualitative evidence. It is what people think has happened, their views and feelings; predominantly of the service user but they could be from, for example, carers or key workers also.

Table 11.4   Key questions of contract review

Reason	Key questions
To ensure or improve quantity and efficiency	Has the provider(s) delivered the agreed service? If not, why not? Is service delivery efficient?
To ensure or improve quality	Is all, most, some or none of the service purchased of an acceptable/satisfactory quality, i.e. does it meet contractual quality standards?
To ensure or improve effectiveness	To what extent has the service achieved agreed outcomes for individuals/the whole service? Why does the service not achieve or only partly achieve some/all outcomes?
To ensure smooth operation of the contract	How do day-to-day working relationships promote or impede the effective operation of the contract? Does anyone have difficulties fulfilling their roles and responsibilities under the contract, particularly because of system and/or communication problems?

In terms of methods of collecting data there are a whole range which will depend on the outcome as well as the time and resources available. Practically there would be a selection from this list of sources due to the constraints of time and money to collect and analyse.

In the example, Figure 11.4 shows the results when residents were consulted about their experience of moving into and living in an extra care housing scheme. The evaluation report focused on achievement of the service outcomes as opposed to individual outcomes. The scaling of results gave scores for various factors as to whether contract outcomes were being met, partially met or not met and were combined with other performance data (e.g. around staff development and training, complaints, etc.) to give a graphic overall picture for the contract.

Strategic level – use of resources, population and benchmarking

At a strategic level one of the most important approaches to measure impact is explored by the Department of Health report *Use of Resources in Adult Social Care* (2009). This document sought to present evidence of what works around prevention, early intervention and personalisation. It urged commissioners to look at the pattern and spend of services and draw conclusions about the nature of investment, particularly for residential care.

This is primarily a comparative or benchmarking approach to services looking at why there is variation between similar services. It is attempting to get to understand why there is difference and, through an analysis of those reasons, find out if a service can be more effective and cost efficient.

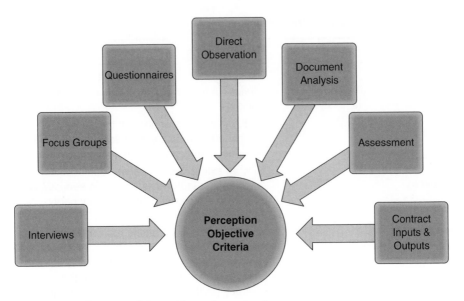

Figure 11.3 Sources of the evidence in contracts

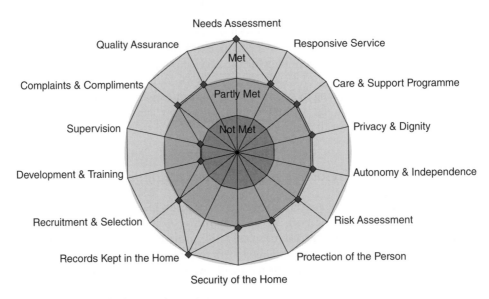

Figure 11.4 Monitoring service outcomes

Source: Department of Health, 2009

For example in the report (DH, 2009) a sample of Local Authorities were chosen and their figures compared for older patients discharged from hospital to residential care. The results showed that there was huge variation between the different areas – which in turn raised questions about the effectiveness of local domiciliary services and assessment systems in keeping people in the community.

This work has been elaborated further by IPC using an 'Investment Model' (Bolton and Kerslake, 2011) which advocates that standard data sets can be useful if combined with commissioners challenging to ask 'the right question' to help understand the current effectiveness of provision and resources.

For commissioning organisations at a strategic level, the purpose of such an approach in a stringent financial climate is to identify mechanisms that manage (or even reduce) demand in the public care system, and to ensure that the optimum outcomes can be delivered with the effective use of resources.

Recent work with a number of IPC Partnership Programme authorities has focused on analysing financial and performance data to improve understanding of the effectiveness of resource utilisation. Above all else the model advocates the need for a solid baseline of data against which the impact of any changes can be considered. It is also suggested to commissioners that judgements about single services are not always helpful – the more challenging and revealing task is to explore the impact of a service against the impact it has on an overall system, e.g. looking at reablement and its impact on the use of domiciliary home care.

Therefore, a key challenge for organisations has to be to identify the relevant performance intelligence (including financial, demographic, market intelligence, contracting and client data) and put in place a performance framework that measures whether the network of services are achieving their required strategic outcomes. For example, each service (whether commissioned from an independent provider or run in-house) should have a clear set of objective measures against which it should be judged on a month by month basis. The service should be reviewed according to these agreed outcomes and changes made if the desired outcomes are not being achieved. The aim of such a performance management framework is to help organisations interrogate data and develop more effective monitoring for the future with an aim of delivering the most effective possible use of resources. As John Bolton has written in recent regional analyses for IPC local authority clients:

> The key message for this work is that we have to robustly challenge ourselves and reconsider our past practices. We have to examine the data available to us with fresh eyes and be open to consider alternative approaches. Most of all we have to break the shackles and limitations of past performance frameworks that have had too many perverse indicators and focus on a new set which are much more focused on outcomes and much less in process.

An example of this outcome focus is shown in Table 11.5 looking at measures for a policy outcome on community impact and older people's independence.

For all public sector commissioners there is a tension about what to benchmark their provision against.

Table 11.5 An example of strategic outcome measures

Policy aim (outcome) – to ensure that the social care system is set up in a way that does not bring people into the state supported care system when there are alternatives that could help an older person retain their independence

Area	Measures	Performance comments
Community impact	The total number of older people in the population whose services are funded by the local authority per 100,000 of older people. The total spend per 100,000 on the older people's population, broken down into: service provision, direct payments, and voluntary sector grants.	There are two aims here: (1) To be able to plot over time and against a comparator group the spend per 100,000 of the relevant population; (2) to be able to measure whether the spend in the voluntary sector on community provision is effective.
	The relationship between outcomes you expect voluntary organisations to deliver, their achievement and level of spend.	Councils need to have the capacity to add grant funding to the amount of direct payments/ personal budgets spent in the voluntary sector to obtain a realistic view of total spend on preventative interventions.
	Numbers of self-funders who run out of capital and move to state support.	
	Total spend on carers in relation to total spend on residential care. Distribution of funding spent on carers.	Effective spending on carers should reduce demand for residential care rather than simply offer a uniform level low level of support to all carers. However, to target spending means being able to identify which elements of carer breakdown drive higher social care expenditure.
	Volume and type of interventions people receive prior to coming into residential care.	A lot of services might indicate that perhaps current provision is not working; no interventions could indicate targeting the wrong populations.
	The proportion of admissions facilitated by the council where the person was not previously known to adult social care.	

General rules would be:

- Measures over time are generally more useful than single snapshots.
- It is vital to be clear about what you are trying to monitor and then testing whether this is the most effective way of achieving that.

- Data capture needs to be easy otherwise the more complex it is then the more likely it is to be error prone.
- It is important to look at whole and interrelated systems. For example, total spend per head of population could go down but spend on the voluntary sector rise. Reablement may displace activity into intermediate care.
- If data is to drive policy, the rate of reporting on items needs to be appropriately set.

Addressing poor performance in contracting

There are two basic approaches to addressing poor performance in services or contracts. How this plays out in reality is often something in-between and will depend on a range of circumstances.

Developmental approach

This starts from the premise that mistakes do inevitably occasionally happen and that everyone should have the chance to learn from them and to change in order to prevent recurrence. Support may be needed to achieve this. In practice the commissioner and provider would agree on what has gone wrong and why. This would be followed by developing a corrective action plan, which may include additional monitoring and/or support for the provider. The contract should make explicit this way of resolving performance problems, and allow eventual termination if satisfactory performance is not re-established.

The benefits of this approach are that it reflects mutual dependence and partnership and can enable 'business as usual' while some matters are resolved. The provider is likely to be positively motivated. The risks are that the provider may think they can 'get away with it' as there are no immediate consequences; the action plan may not resolve the problem and termination may only be delayed not prevented.

Punitive approach

The principle held here is that performance can never be below the required standard. The belief is that financial or other punishments will prevent recurrence of problems; it is also the provider's responsibility to resolve the problem on their own. In practice this would mean the threat or implementation of the reduction of payment or restricting new business or suspension from the accredited list. For these things to happen the contract must contain explicit powers for the commissioner to reduce or withhold payments or restrict new business in specified circumstances.

The benefits of this approach are that there is a very clear relationship between performance and payments and shows the commissioner's serious intent from the outset. The risks are that commissioners can be drawn into terminating the contract sooner than they would want. Judgements to justify decisions to reduce payments or reduce business would be open to legal challenge so the contract must enable the commissioner to take punitive actions.

What determines your approach?

So what would determine a choice of action by a commissioner with a given provider from the two approaches above? Here is a possible set of criteria given by Gosling (2006):

- The seriousness of the matter – where the delivery of the service and/or the quality of care being provided is in question, this will always be more serious than administrative or financial problems. Seriousness will often be linked to risk.
- The risk(s) involved – this will usually be focused on service users, though risks to staff are equally relevant. Another key area of risk is to consider whether the service as a whole is at risk. If closure or withdrawal of registration are possible consequences of the poor performance there are potentially very significant risks for all service users who will need alternative care. Generally, the higher the risks, the more immediate and substantial the response must be.
- Has the contract been breached – has the provider failed to comply fully with the requirements of the contract? When considering poor performance, it is vital to refer back to the contract, to focus on exactly how the provider has not complied with the contract.
- The relationship with the provider – the realities of limited contract monitoring resources and variable provider performance require us to embrace proportionality, i.e. the response

Table 11.6 Two approaches to performance managing contracts (Gosling, 2006)

Developmental approach	Punitive approach
• Mistakes happen. Everyone should have the chance to learn from them and change. Support may be needed to prevent recurrence.	• Performance can never be below required standards. Financial or other punishments will prevent recurrence of problems.
• Purchaser and provider agree on what has gone wrong and why. Develop a CAP, which may include additional monitoring and support.	• The threat or implementation of fine or restriction of new business. Suspension from accredited list. The contract must contain explicit powers.
• Reflects mutual dependence and partnership. Can enable 'business as usual' whilst some matters are resolved.	• Clear relationship between performance and payments. Shows purchaser's serious intent from the outset.
• No immediate consequences for provider – long term deterrent? CAP may not resolve the problem; termination may only be delayed	• Judgements open to legal challenge. Purchaser may be drawn into terminating contract sooner than they would want.

to a high quality provider with very few examples of poor performance would be very different to the response to a poor quality provider with a long history of things going wrong.

- The provider's view and response to the poor performance – when asked about poor performance, a provider may openly confirm where things have gone wrong and show they have or are planning to prevent them recurring. At the other extreme, the provider may either deny there is a problem or, as more frequently happens, provide a series of excuses.

Taking action

It is important in both the commissioning organisation and provider that there is an expectation that managers will respond if poor performance is found – and also how they will respond. Conversations between both sides need to focus on explanation rather than describing problems. If performance is not on target, reports should explain why and what will be done to rectify the problem. The ideal is to achieve a culture in which success is applauded but in which the approach is to minimise the likelihood of failure; if it does occur steps should be taken to ensure that the lessons are learned to prevent repetition in the future.

Improving the operation of a service after identification of a problem will often be about looking at processes and systems, better resources and organisational development – a question here will be how to ensure organisational learning in the provider?

Stop and Reflect

Taking action on poorly performing contracts:

- Remember – monitoring performance alerts you to the fact that a problem exists, not necessarily why it exists.
- Explain rather than describe problems, including how they will be addressed.
- In order to address poor performance you need to analyse reasons behind it and take action.
- Give providers time to analyse and develop a corrective action plan before information is published.

The role of stakeholders and relationships

This book has already discussed how market facilitation is a key function for commissioners. Indeed the Market Facilitation model requires a completely different set of relationships with providers, service users and other stakeholders than the traditional contracting model. Other policy drivers such as personalisation and co-production are also reinforcing these changes. In the traditional model commissioners state what they want and providers deliver according to the contract – the parties tend to be separate with sole responsibilities tending toward fulfilling specified duties in parallel till the end of the contract.

Modern care services, however, are complex, requiring long term planning, high levels of knowledge by the provider and requiring close joint working across agencies to achieve the necessary high levels of service that can be sustained. Commissioners need to have a good understanding of the market and their providers. Figure 11.5 illustrates how relationships are intertwined.

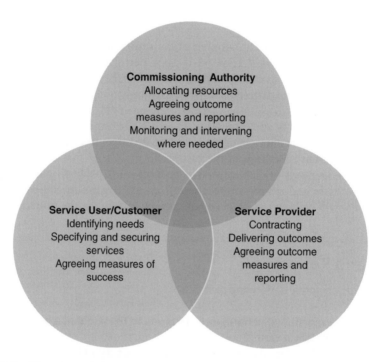

Figure 11.5   Changing relationships

Relationships with providers

We have seen that in setting outcome-based contracts there is greater scope for the provider to focus on delivering the stated outcomes and to be flexible and creative as to *how* these will be delivered. Similarly the commissioner and the provider together would need to agree what are the measures and means of collection for the data to demonstrate that outcomes are being achieved, i.e. the performance management arrangements are a part of a partnership approach. This would include agreement with the commissioners about how service monitoring and evaluation should be constructed.

In terms of contracting processes, Figure 11.6 illustrates how measures in a specification and relationships between providers and commissioners tend to align with the nature of the measures being specified. In other words the requirement for greater

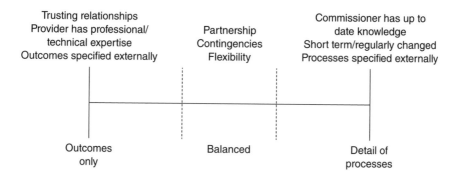

Figure 11.6 Characteristics of contracts and specifications

outcomes goes hand in hand with more long term and trusting relationships between provider and commissioner. Again it is worth stressing that getting the outcomes discussed, agreed and put into the specification with the provider is vital to the future success of the contract. This is one of the most important examples of how the commissioning and procurement parts of the IPC commissioning cycle have to be integrated.

Relationships with service users and carers

At an individual level the same joint approach would apply to the role of service users/carers in the setting of outcomes and how these might be achieved with the associated measures. At a service level, user groups also have a role in the designing and specifying performance arrangements of contracts.

Table 11.7 gives example sources from an IPC client showing outcome performance information for contracts and individual plans that different stakeholders would need to agree.

Table 11.7 Some examples of sources of performance information

Example target	Example measure
Reduction in medication	Medication records
Increase in exercise	Activity charts
Reduction in challenging behaviour	Incident forms
Access to new social/household activity	3rd party verification
Improved contact with family	Self report or 3rd party verification
Increased involvement in running their home	Self report or observation by staff
Improved communication	Self report or observation by staff
Increased involvement in service user meetings	Meeting minutes
Increased engagement in preferred activities	Support plan, shift plans, diaries
Improved daily living skills	Observation by staff, skills checklist

Stop and Reflect

What promotes effective relationships?

- Early engagement with suppliers/providers in developing commissioning strategies and market testing.
- Flexibility about appropriate means of meeting agreed outcomes.
- Open channels of communication.
- Clarity about expectations.
- Transparency of decision making.
- Fair and proportionate specifications and contracts.

CASE STUDY

This case study describes the introduction of the 'Outcome Management' project (Waring, 2006) to measure the impact of Liverpool's spend on adult mental health services. For mental health services in Liverpool the commissioners had set themselves the following ambitious and high level strategic goal: to achieve a community which promotes mental health and prevents the social exclusion of mentally ill people, allowing them to exercise choice, maximise their potential and participate in society safely.

To this end the commissioners determined that all mental health services would be challenged to demonstrate that they were actively contributing to this vision. One goal set by the commissioners was to ensure that all mental health services commissioned by the city council should adopt Outcome Management concepts, methods and tools, irrespective of who was providing those services. The purpose was to target, track, verify and report on the specific health and social gains experienced by service users.

A large number of mental health services were delivered in Liverpool outside of inpatient psychiatric acute services. Some services had been established for many years and were working without any clear service level agreements (SLAs). They lacked explicit goals or measurable objectives against which they could assess how they were benefiting service users.

At the heart of the Outcome Management process was the 'target plan'. Target plans allowed providers to describe the service being provided, and defined service users and performance targets, i.e. changes in the behaviour, condition or satisfaction of service users, including verification methods and milestones for achievement. Templates for each type of service were provided.

In completing their target plan, providers were asked to project the annual gains at each stage on a quarterly basis and were requested to make quarterly returns which were evaluated by the commissioners against the projections in the target plan. Providers were asked to provide explanations for any significant discrepancies between the figures in the target plan and those in the actual returns.

This was not simply a technical exercise involving the commissioners and the providers – service users were at the heart of the process. Service users were in attendance at the seminars, and groups representing service users across the city were, once it had been explained and demystified, very supportive of the initiative. The expectation was that the providers would have an individual target plan for each service user. Where, as an example, a target for a provider was about 'numbers of service users experiencing a mental health gain' this had to translate down to something specific and meaningful for individuals which could be discussed and agreed with each service user.

It was this bringing into focus of the needs of service users which was possibly the greatest benefit of Outcome Management. Support continued to be offered to service providers by telephone, correspondence and through individual visits. Initially, quarterly seminars were held under the title 'Lessons Learned' which enabled both the commissioners and the providers to enhance their understanding of the process.

The move from traditional, often long standing arrangements – whereby financial support in the form of grant aid was passed to service providers in return for an undertaking that they would do 'good things', as evidenced by activity data and annual accounts – to a relationship based on investing for results, was a 'wake-up call' for commissioners, providers and service users alike.

For service providers it meant taking a hard look at their services and realising that they needed to be based on individual plans with individual service users, complete with agreed targets and goals. Rather than engagement between service users and providers being considered sufficient in itself, Outcome Management challenged all to ensure that each activity was purposeful.

The city council and the commissioners of mental health services gained an in-depth picture of the activities which they were funding and were able to improve delivery against some key performance targets as a result of the information provided.

Summary

In this chapter it has been argued that commissioners need to design performance management arrangements systematically and consistently to help them make the best possible judgements about the impact and effectiveness of the services they commission. As we see a greater focus on market facilitation, partnership and mature relationships and on the outcomes that services need to achieve, performance management arrangements are changing and developing.

Further Reading

Walters, M. (1995) *The Performance Management Handbook*. London: CIPD.
Patmore, C. (2002) *Towards Flexible, Person-centred Home Care Services: A Guide to Some Useful Literature for Planning, Managing or Evaluating Services for Older People*. York: SPRU.
IPC (2006) *Commissioning e-book*, CSIP.

References

Bolton, B. and Kerslake, A. (2011) *Models for funding allocations in social care – The £100 million Project*. London: ADASS.

Department of Health (2009) *Use of Resources in Adult Social Care: A guide for Local Authorities*. London: HMSO.

Friedman, M. (2005) *Trying Hard is not Good Enough*. Oxford: Trafford Publications.

Goodspeed, T., Lawlor, E., Neitzert, E. and Nicholls, J. (2009) *A Guide to Social Return on Investment*. London: Office of the Third Sector, Cabinet Office.

Gosling, G. (2006) *Improving Performance Through Effective Contract Monitoring*. Commissioning e-book, CSIP.

Public Private Partnerships Programme (2007) *A Guide to Contract Management for PFI and PPP Projects*.

Triangle Consulting Limited (2006) *The Outcomes Star*. London: London Housing Federation.

Waring, B. (2006) *From Answering the 'So what?' Question: Monitoring Outcomes for Users of Mental Health Services*, commissioning e-book. London: CSIP.

12

Decommissioning

Amongst all commissioning-related activities, decommissioning often attracts greatest public and professional concern. Stories abound about the time spent trying to correct alarmist stories in the local press, disgruntled local councillors fighting the loss of a favourite service in their own wards, and most disturbingly service users and their families left feeling abandoned and unheard amongst a confusing mass of bureaucracy. In a climate of efficiency savings commissioners are often left feeling they are carrying the can for unpopular decisions about the use of resources. However, the process and approach used can mitigate the impact of the changes being implemented

Decommissioning can be a response to a planned change to meet changing needs and expectations of local populations, or to national and local policy drivers including shifting patterns of expenditure, or sometimes it is a response to an unforeseen event, such as the failure of a service in terms of its quality or viability. Whatever the trigger the characteristics of an effective decommissioning process are straightforward:

- Careful preparation.
- Clarity about what you are trying to achieve and why.
- Transparency and good communication.
- Keeping the service user as the focus of the activity.

This chapter looks at these characteristics in more depth, and explores what this means for you as a commissioner drawing on a range of examples to illustrate the main learning points.

Learning outcomes

By the end of this chapter you should be able to:

- Understand what systems and processes need to be in place to support effective decommissioning.
- Be clear about when decommissioning is appropriate, what form it should take and what activities it involves.
- Identify and manage the key risks within the process.
- Develop an approach to communicating with and involving key stakeholders which secures their commitment and minimises the negative impact of change.

Key terms

- *Decommissioning* – the process of planning and managing changes in service, usually either a reduction or a termination, in line with commissioning objectives.
- *Decommissioning policy* – clear guidelines for how decommissioning will be carried out locally which includes the principles or values and also information about local systems and procedures.
- *Communication plan* – a document outlining the responsibilities, consultation structures, governance arrangements, timings and forms of communication necessary when undertaking a project.
- *Managing risk* – assessing risk through looking at the likelihood of an event and the impact it will have, followed by deciding how actively they will need to be monitored, and what you can do to mitigate against them.
- *Impact assessment* – assessing the impact on existing and potential service users, carers, families and the wider population, a consideration of the impact on the provider market and possibly including a diversity impact assessment.
- *Transition plan* – a plan agreed with the provider which takes the service from its current position to the agreed outcome.
- *Change curve* – a model illustrating how people can move through a change process and are likely to respond differently and on an emotional level.
- *Change pool* – a model used to plan effective communication in different forms depending on the purpose and the role of different stakeholders.
- *TUPE* – the Transfer of Undertakings (Protection of Employment) Regulations 2006 (TUPE) protects employees' terms and conditions when a business or undertaking, or part of one, is transferred to a new employer.

When to decommission?

Decommissioning is often seen by those affected as an unplanned response to something outside of their control. This is a natural response to change but there can be a range of factors which lead to the decision to decommission, and it is important to be very clear about which is relevant to the service being considered. Typical factors include:

- Economic circumstances meaning organisations need to review and change their service provision.
- A different response required which addresses the changing needs of the population and the outcomes sought for or by them.
- Recognition of the benefits of alternative service models suggesting changes are needed to existing services.
- A change in demand from service users, particularly with the emphasis on individual choice and control.
- A review of the value for money provided by particular services.
- Quality issues that it has not been possible to resolve in other ways.
- Changes for the provider of the service, such as financial difficulties, or a strategic shift away from this type of service.

You may find that you as commissioner are instigating the change, but equally the drive could be coming from your providers, your citizens or your politicians. The question that needs to be asked is does this change reflect local commissioning intent? Are you able to link the activity back to a written strategy or market position statement (see Chapter 8) which describes local commissioning objectives, resources and approaches? What is the evidence supporting the need to change?

Stop and Reflect

- What factors do you recognise as driving change in services locally? Is it always clear what factors are at play?
- Do they represent or reflect agreed commissioning objectives?

What is decommissioning?

So we understand what might trigger a decision to decommission a service, but what are the options available for you as a commissioner in this situation? What do we actually mean by decommissioning?

Decommissioning is the process of planning and managing changes in service, usually either a reduction or a termination, in line with commissioning objectives. It is not necessarily as clear cut as stopping an entire service completely. It may be that a new service will replace what has been taken away, or the existing service will be changed in some way.

However, it is a process of change, and as such needs setting out and managing carefully. A clear model of how it works for you locally will make it much easier when you are presented with decommissioning as an option.

Stop and Reflect

- Do you have a local definition and description of decommissioning?

But it is also a process which impacts on people and organisations, often significantly, and you will need to be aware of a complex range of competing interests and demands. Poor decommissioning can have wide ranging implications from destabilising a provider market to actually increasing costs; from having a negative impact on vulnerable service users to undermining long term system redesign. So it is helpful to agree a set of principles for decommissioning locally to ensure everyone involved in the process is working to an established approach.

Table 12.1   Developing decommissioning principles locally

Principle	Tests
Transparency and fairness	Do all stakeholders share an understanding of why a decision has been taken to decommission a particular service? Is there fairness in the way different stakeholders are treated, whether between different providers, or different service users?
Welfare of service users	Is safeguarding the welfare of service users a key priority throughout the decommissioning process? Is an essential or important service provision for an individual going to be affected and how is this going to be managed?
Welfare of staff	Is the process transparent for staff affected? Have commissioner and provider worked together to protect the welfare of staff?
Value for money	Is the purpose to ensure that services most effectively meet the needs of vulnerable people, are of the best quality and offer value for money?
Managing risk	Is there clarity about the risks involved, and are they being managed and monitored appropriately?
Partnership	Is there a strong partnership relationship with providers in place already? Is there a partnership approach to managing the process across all stakeholders? Are there particular groups who are not being appropriately involved?
Communication	Has a thorough communication strategy been developed which considers the needs of all stakeholders including service users, staff, elected members, providers and the media?

- Think about what would be important for you as a commissioner in a decommissioning process? What is likely to make you feel it has been a good process? Write a list of these, and then do the same as if you were a member, a provider, and a service user.
- What are the themes running through each list? What is most important? What is the most difficult to deliver?

Preparing for decommissioning

As with commissioning activity more generally it is easy to be unrealistic when decommissioning and to think that a big problem can be solved quickly and without fallout. It is also all too easy to fall into the trap of knee jerk reactions to service failures when caught unawares by problems.

You can help avoid these issues through ongoing performance management of services, an understanding of the provider market locally, and through preparing for the need to decommission. The first two of these are covered in more detail elsewhere in the book, but here we will look at the preparation needed locally to ensure decommissioning is as smooth as possible, and most likely to achieve the outcomes being sought. This is not about individual service reviews, but about the environment within which decommissioning decisions will be made.

A decommissioning policy

Example: A decommissioning policy

An authority is seeking political approval for the decommissioning of a range of community services. In the context of previous feedback about the length of papers received by members, the officer concerned keeps the paper brief but this means that the implications of the review including political sensitivities are not fully explored. In addition, the status of the paper is switched from being confidential to being open without advance notice to the officers concerned and without therefore enabling sufficient time to prepare for the review becoming public to providers, service users and staff.

What would you do differently to prepare the ground for decommissioning activity to prevent this happening? For example what needs to done about:

- Governance arrangements?
- Communication with members?
- Expectations around content of reports?
- Standards for consultation?

There needs to be clear guidelines for how decommissioning will be carried out locally which include the principles or values and also information about local systems and procedures. This is likely to take the form of a decommissioning policy and should have both corporate and political ownership and support. It will include:

- Guidelines on the approach to decision making.
- Risk assessment and management.
- Project management approaches and structures.
- Communication plans.
- Support available to commissioners.

Commissioners need to ensure that they are equipped to undertake decommissioning by being familiar with their local policy and procedures, and also having the expertise and resources to effectively project manage the process.

Contractual relationships

EXERCISE 12.2

Your authority externalised its care homes some years ago, and entered into a 25 year contract with a single provider which included the refurbishment and/or replacement of the care homes. However, more recently demand for care home beds has changed, with more emphasis on people being supported to remain in the community, and the growing popularity of supported housing options. The original contract had not allowed for this or provided an appropriate exit strategy.

- What would you do to prevent this happening with future contracts?
- What would you do to address this situation in the current circumstances?

Initial contract discussions and negotiations with service providers are the ideal time to put in place not only clear service specifications, but also the mechanisms for managing any changes in the future. This should include formally agreed criteria and a framework for possible future decommissioning.

But this is not sufficient. Providers need to be included in regular discussions about their services, the outcomes they are delivering, and future policy direction. This will enable them to plan to meet the implications of any policy changes, and it will also enable you to tap into their knowledge of their service users and potential service users. Your role as commissioner is to build a mature commissioning relationship with your providers, moving away from the adversarial or passive, to a more constructive co-productive approach.

In the example given above, the commissioner was able to change the delivery of the contract to meet local needs all through making best use of an existing close working relationship with the provider and co-producing the solution. This enabled a shift towards extra care housing, and some innovative work with health to make alternative use of some of the existing beds.

Communication

EXERCISE 12.3

You are reviewing a joint alcohol treatment service.

- Who will be the key stakeholders during this review process and any potential decommissioning?
- What existing consultation mechanisms do you have locally that you can tap into? How would you find out about them?
- Do you know the local approach to communicating with the media?

Any changes to service provision will affect and will need to involve a number of different stakeholder groups (see Figure 12.1).

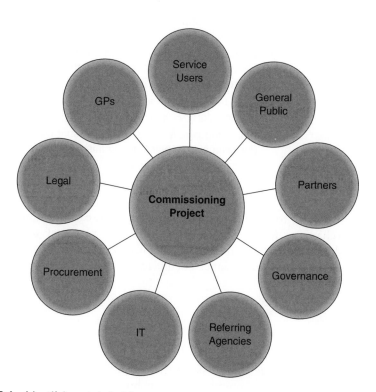

Figure 12.1 Identifying stakeholders

Table 12.2　Developing a communication plan

Topic	Issues that may be covered
Responsibilities	• Who is responsible for communication at particular stages of the process?
	• Who is responsible for liaising with the different stakeholder groups (for example is there one person or team responsible for liaising with the media)?
Consultation structures	• What formal structures are in place for consulting with service users? How representative are they?
	• What provider forums are there, who attends them and what level of engagement is there with them?
Governance	• Who is the appropriate elected member, and what is the best approach with them?
	• What form of communication is best and in what circumstances? When is a verbal report sufficient, and when is a written report necessary?
Timing	• At what point in the process should consultation take place for each stakeholder group?
	• How often should information be given to particular groups? Is it a one-off briefing or ongoing and regular communication?
Forms of communication	• What forms of communication should be used in different circumstances, and depending on the needs of the different stakeholders?
	• What resources are available locally to support this process (for example, translation services)?
	• What language is to be used to ensure clarity of message (for example the word 'decommissioning' can sometimes have incorrect connotations)?

It is not only helpful to be able to identify these groups easily, but also to under-stand local mechanisms for consulting with them. It is very easy to reinvent the wheel so you should try to have information readily available perhaps in a commu-nication plan or some form of guidance document.

Managing risk

There will be a number of risks associated with instigating service change, and you will find it easier to manage these risks if there is a risk matrix template readily available, with guidance for commissioners on how it is to be used. These can become very complex, but the intention should be to ensure they are accessible and effective in supporting the identification and management of risk on an ongoing basis throughout the decommissioning process. Remember managing risk is not a one-off exercise as you need to check progress, and update plans as you work through the process.

Typically risks will be assessed through looking at the likelihood of an event and the impact it will have (see Figure 12.2). Once you have identified where the risks sit within the matrix you then need to decide how actively they will need to be monitored, and what you can do to mitigate against them.

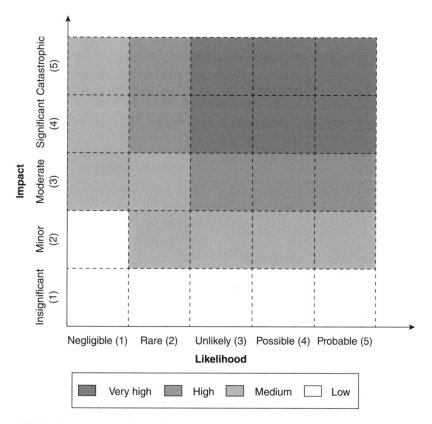

Figure 12.2 An example risk matrix

You are reviewing day services for older people which are currently provided by a number of small providers, as well as one in-house service.

- What are the key risks you will need to manage through the process?
- What is the effect on the provider?

(Continued)

(Continued)

- What is the impact on other services?
- How will this impact on the service users and to what extent?
- Will this affect the working relationship between the provider and the Council?
- Will this alter the current market place?
- What will be the impact of doing nothing?

Making a decision

Rarely will there be just one reason for considering the decommissioning of a service, and the reasons will often include a mix of strategic and operational (see Table 12.3)

It is important to be very clear about the factors at play at the start of the process as this will impact on the direction taken, and the effectiveness of any communication about the decision and subsequent process.

Table 12.3 Identifying decision factors

Strategic factors	Operational factors
A move away from institutional care towards home-based services	Poor outcomes being achieved for service users
A shift in the use of resources across the local authority	Inability of the service as currently configured to meet demand
The withdrawal of national funding for a particular range of services	Poor value for money
Falling demand from service users for this type of service	Lack of sustainability of the service
Withdrawal of support from funding partners	Financial problems for the provider
	Provider withdrawal from the market

Options for change

You will also need to be very clear about what the end game is – what is it you are trying to deliver as a response to the factors you have identified? What are the outcomes for the service user, the provider and the commissioning authority? What does evidence suggest should be the most effective service response?

Just as there are a number of reasons for looking at a service, there is more than one response possible:

- Disinvest or decommission
- Remodel the service
- Renegotiate or end the contract

- Maintain the contract
- Commission new services

Whenever the decision to decommission something is being made, it might be helpful to think through and plot where services are against key criteria (see Figure 12.3). So, for example, how well does the service align with the needs of the target population, set against the quality of the service provision?

Alternatively you could look at the level of risk against the value for money or maybe the impact it provides (see Figure 12.4).

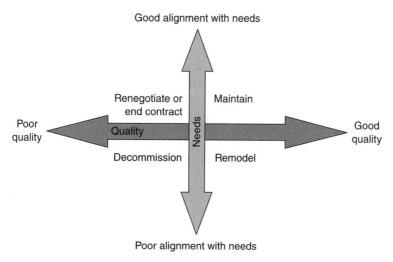

Figure 12.3   Assessing services looking at needs and quality

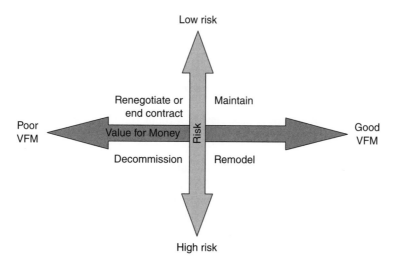

Figure 12.4   Assessing services looking at risk and value for money

There may be other criteria you would wish to use to explore the right option, but there are a number of clear principles which need to be applicable in all cases:

- Be sure about the evidence for change, and be confident it is legitimate and robust.
- Understand what services are actually required to address the needs and expectations of current and future service users, and how the current service compares with this.
- Understand what resources are available, and whether any resources released through the decommissioning process can be recycled into any reconfigured services.
- Engage and communicate with all key stakeholders during the decision process.

CASE STUDY

This case study describes the approach taken by a Primary Care Trust to shift the emphasis of a musculoskeletal service from hospital-based surgical interventions to community-based primary care services without actually decommissioning a specific service. It demonstrates that there are alternative approaches which can be taken when a change in service delivery is required.

The community-based services were focused on remedial interventions which attempted to use 'holistic' approaches to the whole person and a range of treatments including pain care, physiotherapy, exercise and acupuncture. The aim was to remove the need for surgery wherever possible.

There were a number of drivers for the change, including:

- Evidence that surgical solutions didn't always lead to improved outcomes as reported by service users/patients.
- An ageing population and therefore potentially increasing demand.

The key challenges at the outset were:

- The need to shift the behaviours of GPs away from referring patients for surgery.
- The need to persuade hospital consultants and their Hospital Trusts that this different approach was beneficial for patients, effective, clinically safe, and any resulting changes to the business of the Trust could be accommodated.
- The need to stimulate change in the market place through attracting new players and/or partnerships.
- The challenge of attracting new players without contractually decommissioning existing hospital based services.

It was decided that the existing services would not be decommissioned, but instead a new community-based service would be commissioned. The model for the new service was well tested elsewhere but was new to the locality. It was also recognised that given the complexity of the interests at play in the service change, time would need to be spent testing out the new service and developing new care pathways and patterns of referral. As the impact of the new service was understood it would be possible to commission more and to consider decommissioning hospital-based services as appropriate.

The new service is very popular with its users and is seen to be both accessible and effective. The community engagement undertaken for this service change has had beneficial effects: for example, GPs as clinical commissioners now understand the value of gaining support for change from a range of community leaders. However, there are still a large number of patients who are referred direct to hospital-based services. It is not possible to argue that the community-based service has been a substitution for hospital services; however, there have been a number of effects noted:

- Whilst there continues to be an increase in demand for hospital services, this has not been to the degree experienced elsewhere in the region.
- The introduction of the 18 week target time (Referral to Treatment) has had a major impact on orthopaedic services, both in demand and supply. There is evidence that demand for private services has diminished as the waiting time is perceived as more acceptable. Hospitals have had to improve their initial assessment processes and productivity.
- Changing economic circumstances are likely to have impacted on the number of people able or willing to access private health care, thus adding to overall demand for NHS services.
- The range of providers of NHS services continues to grow with new players entering the market through greater use of open procurement mechanisms.

The key lessons drawn from this case study are:

- More time should have been spent at the start bringing key stakeholders on board with the process, and preparing for the impact of their behaviours on the success of the project. This was particularly true of the existing providers and the need to improve their understanding around the outcomes sought, and to plan for conflicting priorities for their staff.
- A more overt use of the clinical pathway demonstrating the desired outcomes for the new model may have assisted GPs in giving more unequivocal support.
- Community engagement was key to the successful implementation of this new community-based service.
- The whole process has taken significantly longer than expected – this was due to the resistance of existing providers to the changes and operational difficulties for the new provider in 'gearing up' rapidly for a new service delivered on multiple sites.
- There was a lack of understanding about procurement processes, and managing contracts amongst some key stakeholders which impacted on their engagement in the process.

This case study demonstrates the impact different stakeholders can have on a project, and the need to ensure this is planned for.

Stop and Reflect

- If you were starting this project, what would you do differently?

Engagement in the decision-making process

One of the challenges you will face is the level of consultation about the decommissioning decision, particularly among existing service users. Sometimes it is helpful to differentiate between the consultation on the decommissioning decision itself and consultation on what individual service users want in the future. What is important is to be absolutely clear at the start about what decisions need to be made, what have been made, and what is open to discussion and debate.

EXERCISE 12.5

Analysis has shown that respite beds in your local area are not being used efficiently with only 55%–60% occupancy despite apparent demand from carers for respite services. An 'in principle' decision has been taken to review the service, and you have taken the information about usage to your Carers Group. The Group are worried that yet more money is going to be taken away from carers services and think the final decision has been taken. They think they are going to be left without any support. The providers have heard about what is happening and have said they are worried about the future viability of their homes because of this threat to their income.

- What could you have done to prevent this situation?
- What could you do to rescue your position with both carers and providers?

In the example above, after the initial reaction of the Carers Group more effort was put into understanding exactly what services were wanted by carers, and what services were being provided by the care homes. Eventually some of the money going in to pay for respite beds was diverted so that a choice could be offered to carers. In addition, more regular communication was set up with both the Carers Group and the care home provider group.

The provider relationship

A number of the examples given have illustrated the importance of engaging early on with the current provider, whether they are from the voluntary sector, the private sector or a statutory provider. You will find that often providers are already aware of issues with the service, understand the needs of service users (both existing and future), and have ideas about alternative service models which will meet the needs of the population and your aspirations as commissioner. An early discussion with the provider will also support any transition required in the future if a decommissioning decision is taken. As has been explored elsewhere, the development of a mature commissioning relationship with providers and a good understanding of the local market, is a key part of your role as commissioner, and will have a significant impact on your effectiveness, particularly when working through a decommissioning process.

There are also contractual implications which could impact on the decision process.

- Does the contract make provision for decommissioning and set out an agreed process?
- Does the contract allow for renegotiation?
- Is the contract nearly at its end, and would it therefore be more appropriate to allow it to run its course, and then transfer or transform the service offered?
- Have terms of the contract been broken allowing for it to be terminated?
- What will be the financial and non-financial cost of terminating the contract early?

You will need to check this when you begin to look at a particular service, but you should also build this in to the design of any future contracts as it can create problems where contracts inhibit the redesign of services.

The decommissioning process

So you have reached the point of needing to move ahead with the decommissioning process, with the necessary agreements in place and a clear idea of what needs to happen. How do you actually take this change process forward?

Project management

As has been described, decommissioning a service is a complex process with a range of potentially competing interests at play. You will need to make sure you have a

Table 12.4   Developing a project plan

Checklist for a project plan	
√	The approach to understanding what existing service users and their carers need from future services.
√	A communication plan for staff, service users, elected members and other stakeholders, including clarity about how consultation will be carried out, and where there is scope for influence and change.
√	A financial plan which includes the costs associated with decommissioning, and how any resources released during the process will be re-used.
√	A review of any contractual issues relating to the service itself, buildings and physical assets, and staff.
√	Transitional arrangements for when the service is decommissioned, which include consideration of any safeguarding and data protection issues.
√	A risk assessment for the process which highlights significant risks and the mitigating action to be taken to minimise them.
√	An overview of the decision structures, project management arrangements including resources, and key milestones.

project plan in place early, with the resources identified and available to manage the process and deliver the outcomes.

You have been asked to carry out a review of low level services for older people and younger adults with physical disability or sensory impairment. This includes both grant-funded services largely provided by small voluntary sector providers, and a long standing contracted service – there are more than 60 providers involved. The intention is to make efficiency savings, modernise contractual arrangements and address the choice and control agenda.

- What approach will you take to project managing a review of this scale?
- What do you think the main issues will be?
- Draft an outline project plan setting out the key milestones.

As you develop a project plan there are some key questions to ask yourself:

- What is the scope of the project, and can it be broken down into smaller projects to ensure it is deliverable?
- Does the project have corporate and political ownership?
- Who is the project manager, and who is the sponsoring officer?
- Is there access to appropriate decision-making powers for the duration of the project?
- Will the project manager be able to take the project through from start to finish?
- Are the timescales realistic? What scope is there for flexibility with the key milestones?
- What is the impact of any legal requirements (such as contractual issues) on the project?
- What communication is needed, with whom, and at what stages?

Impact assessment

In addition to the risk assessment, an assessment of the impact of the decommissioning activity should be carried out now, if it has not already been included in the decision-making process.

This will help you to mitigate the negative impact particularly on more vulnerable groups within the population, and will include thinking about the impact on existing and potential service users, carers, families and the wider population.

This may include a diversity impact assessment or, depending on local practice, this may be a separate and distinct activity.

The assessment will also include considering the impact on the provider market, and particularly whether it will impact on the ability of the market to provide other services. It is important you think about the whole system even when looking at a relatively small part of it in terms of actual decommissioning.

> ## Stop and Reflect
>
> - Looking at the review of low level services considered in the exercise above, what would be the main issues you would expect to see reflected in an impact assessment?
> - What might be the mitigating actions you would include in your project plan?

Working with the service provider

You will have been involving the service provider (or providers) as you have worked through the process so far, but once a decision has been made to enter into a decommissioning process you will need to notify the provider formally. There may be contractual requirements which will need to be considered here, but you also need to be able to work with the provider through a transition period and good working relationships will be key.

The information to be included in a notification would usefully include:

Table 12.5   Developing a transition plan

Content of a transition plan	
Service standards	This sets out the agreed service standards to be met as the service goes through transition, and seeks to protect service users.
Timescale	This will provide clarity about the timescale you will be working to, and what flexibility there is within this.
Information sharing	You will need to seek agreement about sharing and if necessary transferring information with the local authority and any new service providers. This is often difficult to achieve in practice and so needs early discussion to minimise disruption for service users.
Review of process	Regular meetings should be scheduled between the authority and the service provider during the decommissioning process.
Staffing	This will need to set out arrangements for staff involvement and/or redeployment as required, including the need for TUPE.
Media	It is a good idea to have agreement at an early stage about how media communications are to be managed between the authority and the provider.
Contractual arrangements	As applicable there may be contractual issues to be resolved, such as a financial settlement at the conclusion of the contract.

- Advice of the formal decision to decommission the service.
- The proposed period of notice on the contract.
- Information about any appeal procedure and a formal statement that this appeal period has commenced.
- Details of other organisations and individuals to be informed.
- Advice on dealing with any new referrals to the service provider.
- The name and contact details for the officer responsible for the decommissioning process.

You will also want to develop a transition plan with the provider which takes the service from its current position to the agreed outcome.

However, whilst the planning and formal activity is important you need to recognise that you are affecting a change process that will impact on people, who are likely to respond differently and on an emotional level. It can be helpful to be aware of the different responses you may encounter. Figure 12.5 shows an example of a change curve illustrating how people can move through a change process.

So if you cannot get people on board with what you are trying to achieve, the project is unlikely to achieve its desired outcomes.

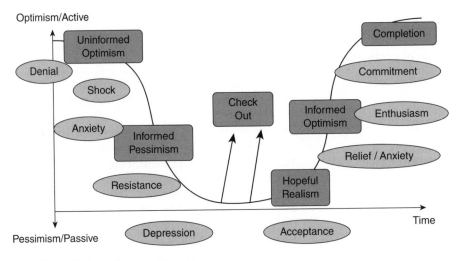

Figure 12.5   Responding to a change process

EXERCISE 12.7

A local authority has been providing short break respite services for children and young people with disabilities for a number of years. The service has been provided by two residential care centres and a staff group of approximately 20, both of which are managed by the local authority. As part of a comprehensive commissioning exercise, the local authority identified the following drivers for change:

- A very small proportion of local children in need who are disabled can access these high cost services.

- Whilst families currently accessing these residential-based short breaks were very satisfied with the service, a much broader base of families would like to see a more flexible offer from the Council, including increased access to home-based care and opportunities for the children or young people to access sport and leisure activities.
- Compared with other alternatives, residential care does not provide good value for money.

The local authority has decided to decommission its residential provision and re-invest in a range of alternative services including more specialist home-based short break services (both in the child's home and with paid short break carers), and more person-alised packages of care including direct payments to families. There is a plan to close the two residential homes but not yet a ready market for the kinds of services the local authority has in mind as a result, including accessible sport and leisure opportunities, personal assistants, specialist short break foster care and other peripatetic carers.

- How would you plan to work with current services to implement this change?
- What reactions could you expect from staff and service users?
- What activities could you undertake to help the process?

Ensuring good communication

We have already discussed the need to plan ahead for communication, tapping in to existing structures and consultation activities, and identifying the key people you will need to involve in different ways.

You will need to think about a number of questions:

- Who may have an interest in this decommissioning process?
- What form of communication will be most effective and in which circumstances? How can you tailor your communication so it is meaningful for the different audiences?
- How often is proactive communication needed and how will you respond to specific issues as they crop up?

You are about to decommission a number of intermediate care beds in a residential care home which have been jointly funded by the local authority and NHS. The care home itself is situated in a small village where it is the only resource locally for older people. It is owned and managed by a small local charity.

Who is likely to need what forms of communication? Consider the change pool shown in Figure 12.6, and use this to tailor your communication depending on where stakeholders fit.

Remember there are different forms of communication depending on the purpose: is it to provide information, to get feedback, to seek agreement, or is it part of working together? Will a newsletter be sufficient, or is individual discussion needed? When would a focus group be appropriate?

EXERCISE 12.8

(Continued)

(Continued)

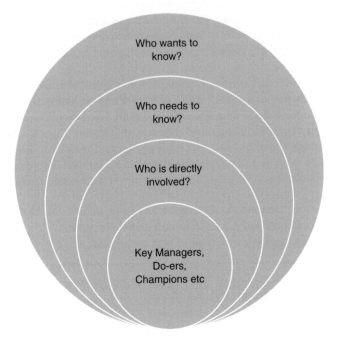

Figure 12.6   Understanding what communication is needed

Having identified the key stakeholder groups above, use the table below to map out what form of engagement is appropriate for each, and therefore what type of communication is appropriate.

Engagement	Stakeholder group
Communication – providing information	e.g. local village population – newsletter every 2 months
Consultation – getting feedback	
Negotiation – seeking agreement	
Participation – working together	

Learning the lessons

As with all commissioning activities you will want to check back on how well the decommissioning process has worked, and to make sure any lessons learnt are shared with others.

This review should include the main stakeholders in the process as far as possible, so service users and/or carers, the service provider, local authority staff, and elected members are likely to be involved. The review should consider the following questions:

- Was there sufficient preparation for the decommissioning activity, with the right policies and procedures in place?
- Was the decision-making process appropriate and effective?
- Was there the right level of communication at each stage of the process?
- Were any communication difficulties managed effectively?
- Was the project management of the process adequate, and were the right skills and expertise available as needed?
- Was there sufficient support for the process in terms of decision making and resources?
- Did the service contract help or hinder the process?
- What were the main barriers to implementing the process effectively and on time?
- What lessons have you learnt individually as a commissioner about what you need to do differently in the future?

Summary

Working through this chapter and its exercises you will have gained an appreciation of the challenges and opportunities presented when you take on a decommissioning task. It is an activity which directly impacts on people: for service users they may feel they are losing a resource, or are welcoming the opportunity to receive a better service which delivers the outcomes they want; for staff they may be losing their job or transferring to another employer, or alternatively they may see the opportunity to deliver a more effective service by working differently.

For you as the commissioner you will need to be clear what you are trying to achieve through working through this process, and the reasons for doing it. This is an important and expected aspect of commissioning as it is the means of ensuring the right services are available for the right people at the right time.

Further reading and web-based resources

Department of Communities and Local Government (2011) *Best Value Statutory Guidance.* London: DCLG Publications.

Transfer of Undertakings (TUPE): The Transfer of Undertakings (Protection of Employment) Regulations 2006 is available at www.legislation.gov.uk/uksi/2006/246/contents/made

Further guidance and advice is available from Local Government Employers at www.lge.gov.uk/lge/core/page.do?pageId=119763

13

Achieving Value for Money

This final chapter explores both the more traditional and the emerging views about value for money in commissioning public care. Councils and their strategic commissioning partners clearly have to develop their commissioning intentions with an eye on what they can afford to deliver. The amount of money available to procure services is a critical part of the commissioning strategy. A commissioning strategy should have a clear recognition of the resources available to deliver the strategic intentions.

In the first section some approaches and tools are outlined as well as some of the risks that can result when commissioners seek to drive down costs. The chapter then moves on to look at the work undertaken by the Department of Health (2009) through its publication *Use of Resources in Adult Social Care* which outlines a way of obtaining best value through the commissioning of social work interventions in order to reduce costs and get better outcomes for people.

Learning outcomes

By the end of this chapter you should be able to:

- Understand that commissioners should always be clear about the links between the resources that are available to them and their impact on their strategic intentions.
- Understand that achieving low procurement costs can lead to higher overall costs – buying something cheap isn't necessarily best value for money.
- Understand that when a commissioner is procuring a service they should always discuss their options with a range of providers in the market. Those who best understand the cost basis of the market and the impact of particular service models on price and outcome are usually those who already provide services in that market. Always discuss your commissioning intentions with potential providers before going out to tender for a service.

- Understand that using an open approach with providers which focuses on the outcomes that the commissioner wants to achieve from the resources available is the recommended approach. This is a mutual process where providers are also prepared to share their costs and profit margins in an approach called 'open book accounting'.
- Understand that if a commissioner is looking at developing preventive services s/he needs to adopt an 'investment approach' ensuring that the money spent on commissioning the service is being repaid through the outcomes that the service is delivering. This may often mean that the cost of the service is outweighed by the savings being made.
- Consider commissioning for outcomes as the preferred route. This can only be achieved if all other key parties are also working towards outcomes. All assessments should be outcome-focused; all providers should be able to demonstrate the outcomes they are achieving and all service users should be able to see the impact of the services they are receiving in terms of the outcomes achieved.

Key terms

- *Procurement* – purchasing specified services.
- *Tendering* – the process used to purchase services which is usually done through issuing a service specification of what is required and invites those who wish to run the services to bid against each other. The choice of who wins the contract is normally determined by a combination of quality and cost.
- *Outcome* – how a person perceives the benefits or otherwise of a service they have received.
- *Best value* – the term which defines a process which considers the balance between the cost of a service or outcome with the quality of the service/outcome achieved.

Securing best value – approaches, tools and risks

The traditional way in which value for money has been identified has been through a calculation of the quality of a service against the cost of that service. On the basis that many councils are procuring similar services, a simple past measure of value for money was based on the unit costs of services. Councils and their health partners have focused on how to reduce the costs they pay for services and they have used a range of methods to achieve lower prices. The methods are primarily driven by the way in which a service is procured (rather than commissioned). For example:

- Externalising an in-house service through competitive tendering of that service.
- Competitive procurement by encouraging a range of independent providers to compete on price for a service and awarding a tender based on the lowest price (possibly balanced against a minimum quality standard).
- Entering into a procurement exercise as above with neighbouring councils (e.g. the North and South West Wales Procurement Groups, the West London Procurement Group). The aim is to achieve lower costs through higher volumes and lower overhead costs for providers. An alternative approach to joint-procurement is to establish a bench marking club where commissioners share with each other the price they are paying for particular services. It has been found that commissioners may be paying different prices for the same services. Comparing prices paid is a way to avoid this practice as commissioners work with providers as a group to agree a suitable price.
- Entering into a commissioning and procurement process with partners in local health services (Joint Commissioning). There are two benefits identified from councils and health services combining their commissioning functions. First, there are economies of scale where the infrastructure costs of commissioning and procurement can be reduced through a combined team. Second, there is some practice where it has been found that one party can procure services at lower prices than the other, e.g. the price the respective partners pay for nursing home beds. In a number of places the health commissioners have handed over all of the procurement of residential and nursing care beds to councils.
- Stating the maximum price that a commissioner will pay for a particular type of service or a local rate for a set of services – commonly used in residential care for older people. Many councils have set a rate they will pay and in the last couple of years they have not increased that rate (even in line with inflation).
- An alternative to this approach is called a 'Dutch auction' where potential providers are invited to tender for a price which reduces at each stage until the lowest price offered by a provider is then selected as the preferred provider for that service. This approach has been used to procure nursing care but was very unpopular with many providers.
- Using a fair price mechanism that looks to link the price paid according to the needs of the customer – commonly used for adults with learning disability in residential care (and linked to personal budget resource allocation systems).
- Open Book Accounting where the provider is open about how their costs are calculated and the agreed price is then negotiated with those procuring the services based on this transparent information.
- Transfer from a more expensive service provider to a cheaper alternative or closure of an expensive service expecting others in the market to meet any gaps in provision.

In the 1990s significant savings were reported by councils who either closed down their in-house services in favour of issuing lower cost contracts to the independent sector or through councils passing over their existing services direct to an independent provider. Savings were made through a combination of paying lower wages and pensions alongside lower management and support costs. However, subsequent legislation about the transfer of staff to new providers of services has made it much less likely that savings will be generated in this way as both staff pay and pensions are protected when a transfer of employment takes place. There are, however, still examples in residential care and in domiciliary care (particularly in-house reablement teams) where the very high costs of the in-house service might make the transfer or closure of the service an attractive proposition in order to save money.

All of these approaches have been adopted by some commissioning and procurement teams. There are a number of risks associated with driving down the costs about which commissioners should be aware:

- New approaches to how people who come to social care for assistance may lead to higher initial costs of interventions such as a reablement service which can lead to lower overall costs. This needs to be taken into consideration when looking at commissioning strategies.
- Where some services have been procured at a very low cost it is probable that the quality will also suffer. This may have the impact of closing down services as they may not survive external criticism (which may impact on overall supply which then in turn could lead to a shortage which is likely to drive up the price in the long run). It is also possible that low quality services cannot meet a person's needs which actually will mean that the service user will need more of that service which overall leads to higher costs. This has been seen as a phenomenon in domiciliary care.
- In residential care many councils set a maximum price they will pay for the service. In many cases this rate is less than the price calculated by independent sources as being the realistic cost of care. This has led to a situation where older people coming into residential care may be asked to find a third party to pay a top up on the fees required. This is an area which has not been fully examined or tested in the courts. However, recent judgements on Judicial Reviews have demonstrated that care providers will now start to challenge councils where the cost of care has been driven to a low level either through a refusal to offer annual inflation uplift or through other means of keeping the payment by the councils for fees unrealistically low.
- In some areas there is a risk that a focus on price could lead to poorer outcomes. Achieving a low price for residential care could lead to too many people being offered residential care as a solution to meet their care needs when alternatives (which sometimes can be at lower costs) could have been available that would have enabled a person to retain a degree of greater independence which is what many people say they would prefer.
- There is some evidence that integrated health and social care systems actually procure higher cost services than their counterparts who procure separately. This evidence suggests that where health staff have the dominant culture in a joint service, there are likely to be higher levels of admissions to residential care, higher admissions to hospital and higher re-admissions, adding costs to the system. However, where a joint commissioning team has shared objectives with a set of shared outcomes, which include looking to commissioning to achieve lower non-elective admissions to acute hospitals, lower admissions to residential and nursing homes and has made an investment in Intermediate Care, Reablement and Post Hospital Care and Support, then it is more likely that lower overall costs can be achieved and better value delivered.

For all the ways in which commissioners may have to assist them in securing lower costs, one of the best ways to secure value for money is to maintain an open dialogue with each provider. Commissioners must understand the cost pressures born by the provider as well as have an understanding of the factors that will contribute to the price of a quality service. Given that wages generally make up around 30% of the costs of residential care and 60% of the costs of domiciliary care, councils should acknowledge that low prices will equate to low wages which in turn is likely to lead to higher staff turnover, less well-trained workforces and subsequently poorer quality services.

If a council has obtained a lower cost for the service it has procured does this mean that it will have achieved better value? Several factors emerge that have made councils reconsider this 'traditional' approach including the fact that driving down the price does not always produce the outcomes that are expected. This is par-ticularly relevant for domiciliary care where low wage levels and uncertainty over staff contracts gives a very high turnover of staff. The range of prices paid by local authorities for external home care demonstrates that fees paid to independent pro-viders in some parts of the country are not sufficient to provide good quality care (UKHCA, 2012).

It is not only the price that may be of concern to providers of domiciliary care but the United Kingdom Home Care Association's (UKHCA, 2012) recent report was also highly critical of the number and range of hours (or more specifically part hours) that are procured by councils. They reported that pressures on providers are exacerbated because of the demands for prompt hospital discharge and the increas-ingly complex needs of service users. Their study found that 58% of independent providers and 43% of local authority providers responding to their survey reported that more than half the visits they made, as part of a package of care purchased by social services, were 30 minutes or less. 40% of independent providers and 73% of in-house providers reported taking on some visits of 15 minutes or less, in order to check on service users and assist with medication. Independent providers with block contracts were more likely to take on these very short visits than providers with spot purchase contracts. It was reported that older people were more likely than younger service users to receive short visits.

In addition the report highlighted the following weaknesses in the system:

- Communication between care managers and providers in addressing the needs of service users is very variable.
- The closure of cases by care managers is resulting in providers taking greater responsibility for care packages without financial or other recognition by social services departments.
- Providers are increasingly likely to be invited to reviews by care managers.
- The practices of care managers may be inconsistent with the expectations of providers laid down in the National Minimum Standards for domiciliary care.

Earlier in the chapter it was already indicated that there is some evidence to suggest that if one procures domiciliary care at the lowest possible price that this might actually drive up demand for that service which will overall increase the cost of the service. Evidence from national data returns (NASCIS) shows that the increase in demand for domiciliary care hours comes from existing customers not from the increased demands of new customers.

Stop and Reflect

- Beware that reduced price could lead to reduced quality which might in the end lead to higher overall costs.

CASE STUDY

One joint commissioning team wanted to develop new services to help older people who were being discharged from hospital. It decided to invite a wide range of providers to meet with them to explain what the problems were that they faced. After a meeting with a large group of providers they then had 1:1 meetings with about a dozen different organisations listening to how they would address the problems that were identified. As a result of the range of excellent suggestions made by providers the council then felt much more confident in what they wanted to procure. This enabled them to go back to the market for the procurement stage knowing how the problems could be addressed in a way that would not have been possible without the preliminary stages.

EXERCISE 13.1

Consider a piece of commissioning that you are currently undertaking:

- What are the factors that you need to consider between the cost of any future service, the quality of that service and the outcomes that your overall strategy wants to achieve?
- Make a list of your key objectives.
- Make a list of the risks that may emerge.
- Make a list of the potential providers with whom you may want to have a conversation before proceeding to the next stage (formal tendering).
- Which other stakeholders might need to be involved in the process?
- Should this be better done with neighbouring commissioners?
- How will you judge success of the commissioning plan?

Personalisation and commissioning

Earlier chapters in this book have looked at the implications for commissioning arising from the move to increasingly personalised services. In relation to value for money there is some concern that personalisation of services may remove some of the value within the system and lead to higher pricing. This is mainly due to some of the economies of scale achieved through bulk procurement (buying large volumes of the same service) and through seeking to keep down the transaction costs for providers and councils through a simple system of identifying customers who have actually received the service that was procured for them.

The debate about whether personal budgets provide better value is inconclusive. An early study by SPRU (2008) did not find sufficient evidence to suggest that lower costs would necessarily result from the more effective use of resources by service users. Some of the early anecdotal evidence showed that adults with learning disabilities moved from residential care to community-based settings at lower costs to the council, as a result of using their personal budgets to achieve this. There is also some anecdotal evidence that people receiving direct payments may be making lower cost packages of care than they used to receive when their services were directly provided by councils. However, when the associated support costs for people receiving direct payments are taken into account the differences appear to be small.

Councils are still letting out contracts for large volume services such as Domiciliary (Home) Care, supported living and some day and residential care. The aim is to secure a certainty for those services regarding where there is likely to be demand and to secure a reasonable price through the large scale of these services. There are now examples of social enterprises and other new creative solutions that are often part of a very local package of care, which are attempts to keep down these costs.

Overall, there is no convincing argument to suggest that personal budgets will inevitably save a council money. Councils will continue to be required to ensure that there is a supply of services through their area and this may be achieved through market position statements or through some procurement mechanism (see previous chapters). Service users require a good range of services at an affordable cost to their personal budget allocation. Commissioners are still responsible for achieving this on behalf of the majority of customers, including in some cases those who will purchase their own care (self-funders).

Stop and Reflect

- Don't assume that personal budgets inevitably mean lower costs.

Does commissioning from the not-for-profit sector secure better value?

An important question to be considered is whether savings are secured through working with the voluntary sector, social enterprises or other forms of mutuals. Although this may appear on the face of it to be a good way of getting value for money, this is not guaranteed given that the sector covers a wide range of different organisations, funding mechanisms and structures. These may vary from those that are voluntary only in their governance but have full time paid staff and work almost exclusively to state-funded contracts, to those that are wholly voluntary in income and labour. Mutuals vary in size and type from small local cooperatives through to BUPA as a multinational health and care provider. No single structure can be considered automatically good or bad. Even those organisations that are voluntary only in their governance arrangements may still be open to innovation, have lower labour costs due to different working terms and conditions from local authorities, and offer greater flexibility about their approaches to service delivery. They may also enjoy a higher level of public acceptance.

In recent years most local authorities have begun to change their relationship with the voluntary sector, moving from grants to contracts, where there is a defined connection between the fees paid for the service received. Additionally there is increasingly also an expectation that contracts will have a strong focus on outcomes.

New forms of organisation such as Social Enterprises (not-for-profit organisations that use any surplus made to feed back into a community-based project) and Workers Cooperatives are being increasingly encouraged to develop by government policy. Their value depends on well-motivated workers and creative energies to keep and sustain new organisations when resources are scarce for the funding of new enterprises. Some councils are concerned that European procurement rules prohibit them from nurturing such new schemes without using some form of formal procurement.

However, social enterprises that are local authority 'spin outs' are likely to offer something of a mixed benefit. To be successful they may need to initially rely on a local authority block contract (which runs somewhat contrary to personalisation) and be relatively high cost if staff are transferred from the council to the social enterprise under TUPE arrangements. Yet if they are successful they may then be reluctant to work for local authorities if they can attract higher levels of funding from self-funders in an open market.

Stop and Reflect

Though the common feature of 'not-for-profit' organisations is that they are not looking for a return on their investments to satisfy shareholders' or directors' interests they may not necessarily be run in a way that delivers the most cost effective use of resources. Those commissioning services need to do more than 'judge a book by its cover' in order to determine if an organisation is more or less likely to deliver value for money.

Commissioners who are in touch with service users will be looking for feedback from those customers as to the quality and suitability of the services that are being provided at all times. This will mean that from time to time commissioners will receive unfavourable comments from service users about the services which have been commissioned for them. There are two separate issues to consider here. Firstly, always remember that the initial comments are those of a particular service user with a unique set of expectations and experiences. Keep an open mind as to whether the provider is failing all other service users as well or just this one person and whether it is the service provider who needs to improve what they are doing or the service user who needs a different service.

All complaints warrant a level of investigation which should be open and transparent. Contracts for services are legal documents and as such all investigations require the commissioner to follow a proper independent process. Do not make accusations but look into the facts and determine (with legal advice where necessary) if a breach of the contract has occurred and what action is required. In most instances a simple letter explaining what you think has gone wrong and what remedies are required will suffice. Monitoring situations closely, and working with providers and customers to help get things right is a preferred option. Where there has been a serious breach of contract or a service user has been put at serious risk then termination of a contract through a proper legal process is a path to follow.

In some cases providers have bid for contracts at a price where they cannot then deliver the service to the required standard. Of course, it is always best that this is clear before contracts are awarded and it is the commissioner who awards the contracts. This is why determining best value on price alone is not the best way to approach the awarding of contracts. In all cases in the first instance it is best to work with providers to make the required improvements rather than to resort to legal actions which can be both time-consuming and costly themselves. There are examples where commissioners have been prepared to pay more for a service in order to get the required quality of service or outcome for the service users.

Best value through effective investment in the right services

Does low cost equate to best value?

It is important to distinguish between determining the kind of interventions or services that one might commission and the price or quality of those services. The new emerging view on value for money comes from work that is based around three emerging themes:

- Commissioning for outcomes
- Commissioning to get the right interventions that reduce need for state-funded support
- Developing an investment approach to commissioning

All of these themes have at their heart a sense that better value is achieved through an overall reduction in total costs across the whole system rather than a low cost for a specific service, e.g. if a council is only purchasing small amounts of residential care it is likely it will be paying a higher unit cost for each care contract than a council that makes wider use of residential care. However, it is generally accepted that keeping adults or children in their own homes is less expensive than placing people in residential care. There is sometimes a debate around this assertion, but overall the evidence suggests that this is the case (DH, 2009). That is not to say that some packages of care that councils have agreed with their customers are not more expensive in the community. Overall, a council with fewer residential placements is likely to be spending less money per service user. There are a whole range of services that a council may wish to commission if it wishes to reduce its admissions to residential care. These might include a range of intermediate care services for adults:

- Reablement-based services
- Out-of-hospital care
- Short-term recuperative-based residential care

Or a range of interventions to help families stay together:

- Family intervention projects

Or a range of housing-based alternatives to residential care:

- Extra-care housing
- Sheltered housing
- Supported living schemes
- Housing with support for care leavers
- Use of assistive technology
- Use of disabled facilities grants to adapt properties for disabled people including children and their families

All of these services will be commissioned with a view to reducing overall costs through having fewer people in more expensive-based facilities. A short-term investment in a preventive service may reduce overall longer-term costs.

In order to assess whether a set of interventions produces value for money the investment approach to prevention has been developed (ADASS, 2010). This approach simply asks commissioners to look at what they need to spend on a set of interventions and then asks them to calculate if the ensuing savings achieved determine if the investment was worthwhile. So for adults' services, whether an investment in domiciliary care reablement leads to a reduction in demand for domiciliary and residential care or health services, or for children's services whether an investment in family intervention projects leads to reduced spend elsewhere on family services (see, for example, Catch22, 2011).

Figure 13.1 demonstrates the process in adults' social care that many councils have adopted that looks to contribute to the way that the total system is commissioned so that best value is delivered.

The interventions can either support recovery and rehabilitation, offer preventive measures to stop a recurrence of the problem (e.g. falls clinic) or help someone better adapt and live with the problem they have (e.g. programmes that support older people and their carers where there has been an early diagnosis of dementia). This approach on adults' social care has a close parallel in the approaches being taken in

Information and advice (focus on prevention and directing
people to resources outside the formal care system)

Assessment for short term outcome (carried out by
reablement team)

Assessment for longer term outcome (social work
assessment with continued reablement)

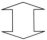

Constant review by providers and by assessors (where
appropriate) of outcomes to be achieved

Figure 13.1   Commissioning best value process

many children's departments to results-based accountability. The simple message is that all interventions should be planned on the basis of improving the outcome for the customer. For many customers this could lead to a better set of outcomes being achieved at a lower long term cost for the state.

Outcome-based approach to commissioning.

Earlier in the book reference has been made to 'outcomes-based commissioning'. This chapter gives an example of this from adults services in a county in England which has moved to a developing model of outcome-based commissioning, including payment by results for their domiciliary care. The focus is on outcomes that help older people promote their independence and in looking to achieve this from their commissioning, the county expects to make further savings.

CASE STUDY

One council wanted to create a single entity which it would call the 'Helped to Live at Home Service'.

The service would be built around the expressed wishes of service users and delivered in relation to the outcomes they wanted, that of helping them move towards greater independence. This would be used as the basis of their definition of personalisation.

The choice of the activities which must be undertaken, that are agreed by the customer, to enable them to deliver their stated outcomes.

The assessment functions would be available for all citizens in the council irrespective of eligibility criteria or ability to pay for a service, i.e. the assessment service would help self-funders.

There would be a good up front advice and information service run by the local authority and easy access to equipment and small adaptations including telecare products. There would be a strong element of housing support and advice within this service (linked to the development of extra-care housing across the county).

Their contracts would be for a limited number of suppliers (with eight district contracts available for tender) and they would aim to pay contractors on the basis of the outcomes they achieved.

In the end the eight contracts were awarded to different suppliers three.

Existing customers could take a direct payment if they wished to stay with their current provider – otherwise they would move to the new contractors.

Staff from the council's domiciliary care services would transfer across to the new providers – including current reablement teams. The new service would not have a separate reablement team as this would become the main approach of all providers.

Assessments for outcomes would be carried out by the assessment and care management teams in the council. Providers would be responsible, with the customers, for determining how then they would deliver the services to meet the defined outcomes with a strong emphasis on using community resources as part of the way to meet the person's needs (desired outcomes). The plans of the providers and the older people would be 'signed off by the Council'. Providers would be paid on the agreed outcomes rather than on any stipulated hours. Penalties would be applied where the failure to deliver an agreed outcome was clearly the responsibility of the provider.

The community-based health services would also look to contract with the same providers. The provider is also responsible for informing the council if they think that a payable outcome cannot be achieved.

The payment would allow for a short period of 'help' whilst the Support Plan is being agreed with the customer. After that initial period the provider will be paid on the outcomes achieved. The customer would receive the first six weeks of care free of charge in line with Government Guidance.

Commissioning for outcomes and paying rewards to providers who deliver purposeful interventions that help reduce dependency on care services and support individuals to live independent lives, must be the future way forward. However, in order to achieve this it is the whole system that needs to change – it cannot be driven by commissioning alone. In particular, Assessment and Care Management staff and social workers need to work alongside service users to establish desired achievable outcomes, and providers must be willing to assist service users in attaining their outcomes through appropriate interventions. There is a general lesson here for all commissioners.

Pugh in her paper on outcomes-based accountability (2010) has the following questions which clearly state what every commissioner should be asking themselves:

1. Who are our users?
2. How can we measure if our users are better off?
3. How can we measure if we are delivering services well?
4. How are we doing on the most important of these measures?
5. Who are the partners that have a role to play in doing better?
6. What works to do better, including no-cost and low-cost ideas?
7. What do we propose to do?

EXERCISE 13.2

Consider an example of the next piece of major commissioning that you need to address in your local area.

- What are the key outcomes that you want to achieve for your customers from this commissioning?
- Have you discussed these with a group of current service users?
- Have you discussed these with assessment/social work staff?
- Have you discussed these with your key partners?
- Have you discussed these with your current providers?
- Can your current providers deliver improved outcomes and lower your overall costs?
- Are there likely to be other providers in the market who could achieve this?
- What do you need to change in order to achieve the desired outcomes?
- What are the likely costs going to be if a different specification is drawn up?
- What are the likely benefits from this new specification?
- Do the benefits outweigh any additional costs?

Another example of investment in services might be an approach to the benefits of using assistive technology.

Technology is currently and is likely to continue to play an important part of any future commissioning strategy. For example, councils will continue to commission community alarms to help older people and some disabled people feel safer in their own homes. (This is seen as being cost effective as it overall costs less than say organising 15-minute visits from a domiciliary care worker to check up that people are doing alright.) The development of new technologies will mean that there will be a range of different pieces of equipment which will service different needs that can assist people in their own homes, from the electronic gadgets that ease life in the kitchen, to those that remind someone to take their medication or ring an alarm when someone is incontinent to help alert a carer to help change the sheets. Newer technologies include monitoring devices that can help track a person with dementia, check that someone is feeding themselves or alert a carer when the front door is opened. The development of new health technologies mean that a person's vital signs can be measured each day and a questionnaire can be completed online which can alert a medical team when someone is at risk and requires a visit. All of these devices will assist in helping people live in the community and will probably reduce both emergency hospital admissions and admissions to residential care. They do, however, need to be carefully and thoughtfully commissioned.

The publication *Models for Funding Allocations in Social Care* (ADASS, 2011) identifies the following way of examining the use of telecare:

- Replacement – The existence of a range of telecare supports means there is no need for the physical presence of care and support staff, e.g. a telecare device could remind people to take their medication.
- Reaction – The existence of a telecare device means that somebody gets a service quicker and hence lessens the need for high cost interventions, e.g. emergency services are alerted quicker if somebody falls over following a stroke.
- Reduction – A cheaper service can be offered because telecare equipment can ensure someone's safety, e.g. discharge from hospital takes place sooner because technological devices can safely support their return home.

It is now possible to add to this list: Reablement, where the gadget can help assist with the delivery of the recovery process and help the customer with the self-management of their condition. In health care the use of monitors for vital signs can ensure that visits to patients at risk can be prioritised and other visits reduced.

It is not the investment in the new assistive technology alone that usually delivers the savings that the investment model suggests. Usually, each of these uses of technology is part of a wider commissioning strategy that is helping older or disabled people remain in their own homes. But the investment in the technology alongside the other services can be judged against the reduction in spend elsewhere to demonstrate improved outcomes at lower costs.

Not all investments in prevention can demonstrate a return. The evidence from a range of literature suggests that prevention is most likely to succeed when it is targeted on specific problems or populations with structured and measurable interventions. In essence there are three tests to be applied across the range of provision in assessing the contribution such targeted interventions might make to people's health and wellbeing:

1. How well can we identify populations who are most likely to benefit from any proposed intervention? Obviously the capacity to predict who will need high intensity, high cost care improves the greater the level of need an individual already possesses. Universal provision may reach a large number of older people but amongst that population it is hard to predict who will go on to need high intensity interventions.
2. At the other end of the scale there may be people who have already had a number of hospital or care admissions, where the goal may be not to avoid high intensity health and social care but to delay its take up. Is there an evidence base which identifies interventions that will work for the population identified and achieve the desired outcomes and is it possible to monitor the impact that they might have?
3. Finally, is the intervention acceptable to the recipient and likely to be followed? For example, community pendant alarms may be a low cost intervention but their success will be limited if their design is unacceptable to service users who may simply choose not to wear them.

Summary

This chapter focuses on value for money. In the first part it looks at the issues when commissioners are looking to reduce the costs of the services they are required to procure and concludes that low costs don't necessarily equate to better value for money. In the second part the issues surrounding commissioning for outcomes and the investment model of commissioning for prevention are considered. The conclusions indicate that best value is achieved through a focus on the outcomes that a contract can deliver for an agreed price. The ability to measure the outcomes and to know the impact that the service has for customers is an important part of the process. In all matters working closely with providers, customers, assessment/social work staff and with partners is critical to achieve the best value to which the commissioner aspires.

References

ADASS (2010) *How to Make the Best Use of Reducing Resources: A Whole System Approach*. London: ADASS.

ADASS (2011) *Models for Funding Allocation in Social Care – 'The £100 Million Project'*. London: ADASS.

Catch22 (2011) *Right Time, Right Support*. London: Catch22.

Department of Health (2009) *Use of Resources in Adult Social Care: A Guide for Local Authorities*. London: HMSO.

Pugh, G. (2010) *Outcomes Based Accountability: A Brief Summary*. London: IDeA.

SPRU (2008) *The IBSEN Project – National Evaluation of the Individual Budgets Pilot Projects*. University of York: Social Policy Research Unit.

UKHCA (2012) *Care is not a Commodity*, commissioning survey. Sutton: UKHCA.

Index